"I love it, we got this! When you are going through it, you are looking for someone that's got you and she does."
  —*ROBIN ROBERTS*, Good Morning America

"Elissa is magic. She has taken the pain and hardship of living with a terminal illness and alchemized it into a zest for life unlike anyone I've ever known. These pages are a peek into her incredible outlook. What a gift."
  —*GRACE HELBIG*, comedian, actress, and *New York Times* bestselling author of *Grace & Style: The Art of Pretending You Have It*

"I love how she says 'prioritize living.' That's the stuff!"
  —*GINGER ZEE*, Good Morning America

"You took this as an opportunity to change other people's time when they're dealing with something terrible."
  —*ARAKSYA KARAPETYAN*, Good Day LA

"The wisdom distilled in *We Got This* is not just a road map for cancer patients, survivors, and the communities that support them. It is a testament to the human spirit and how to live a purpose-filled life."
  —*ANDREW MCMAHON*, from the Foreword of *We Got This*

WE
GOT
THIS.

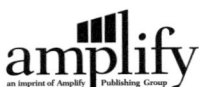

amplify

an imprint of Amplify | Publishing Group

www.amplifypublishinggroup.com

We Got This: How I Learned to Thrive with Terminal Cancer

For more information, please contact:
Amplify Publishing, an imprint of Amplify Publishing Group
620 Herndon Parkway, Suite 220
Herndon, VA 20170
info@amplifypublishing.com

Library of Congress Control Number: 2024922477

CPSIA Code: PRV0225A

ISBN-13: 979-8-89138-354-8

Printed in the United States

To Ellie

If I'm ever not here with you, I hope the pages of this book remind you of how deeply I lived my life, all because of you.

In loving memory of my brother, Josh Slovin

I'm grateful for the bond we shared, for the sibling relationship that thrived in the end. I wish we had more time, but your memory and your heart live on.

To cancer thrivers everywhere

You are not alone. Together, We Got This.

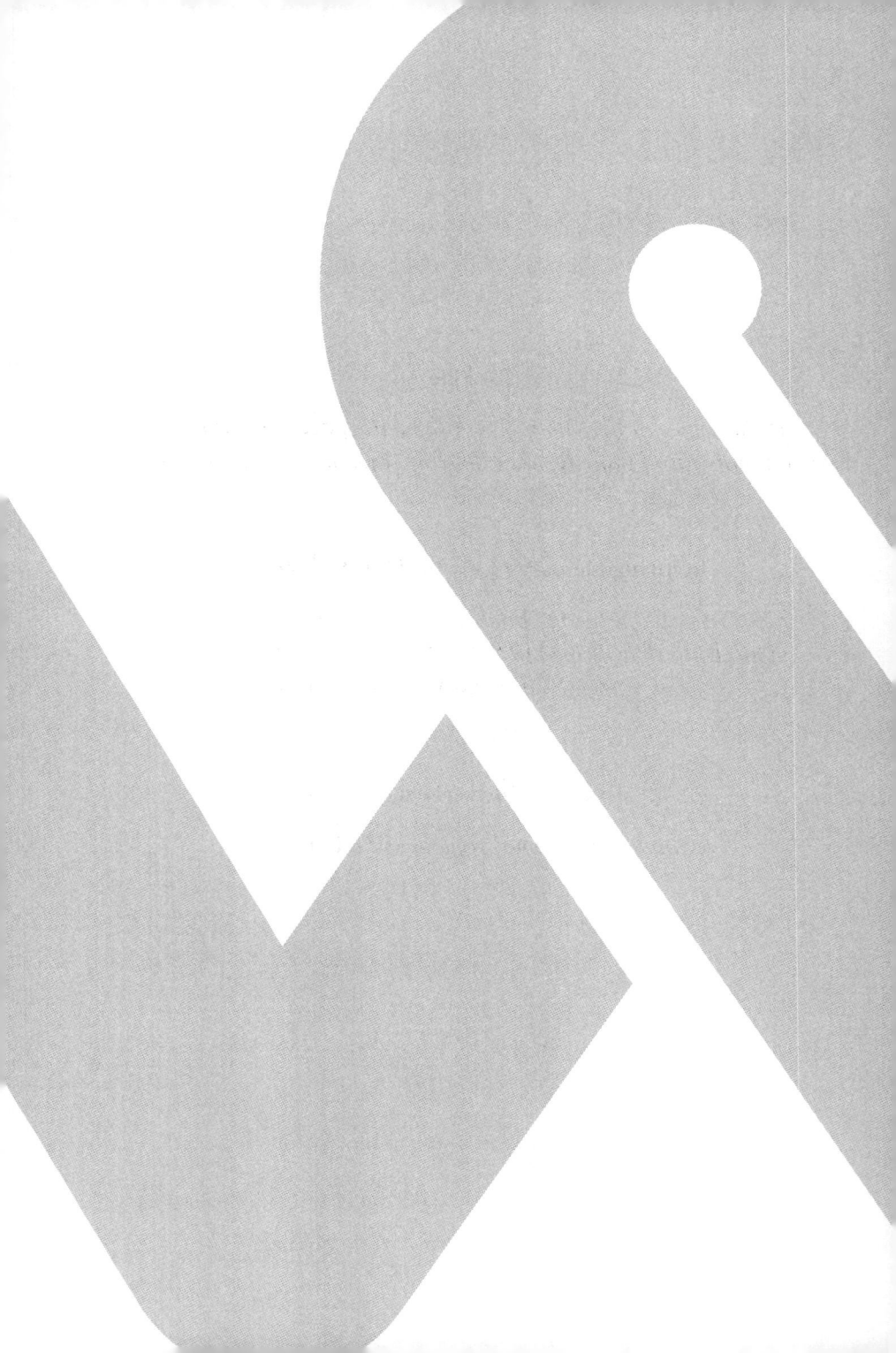

WE GOT THIS.

HOW I LEARNED TO THRIVE WITH TERMINAL CANCER

elissa kalver

amplify
an imprint of Amplify Publishing Group

CONTENTS

FOREWORD

I met Elissa Kalver on a rooftop in Detroit at the end of a three-day public speaker's conference. It was a cocktail party, the last big event of the weekend, and I think everyone was glad to have a moment to enjoy each other's company and reflect on what we'd learned. I say everyone, but I'll admit I did not count myself in that cohort. It's not that I didn't enjoy the conference—I did, but I am not yet a public speaker and I was there mostly as a fly on the wall, listening to the incredible stories of the other attendees and gaining insight on how one might make a career in speaking.

Despite being a performer and public figure, I find gatherings with strangers overwhelming and am terribly self-conscious when making small talk. I did what I do in those situations: grabbed a drink and found a spot in a corner and tried to make myself invisible. One of the hosts of the event clocked what I was up to, kindly grabbed a seat at my high-top table, and began scanning the space. She didn't want me to miss an opportunity to network with this admirable group whose stories and perspectives have been tapped to inspire and transform lives. Less than thirty seconds passed before she had grabbed me by the arm and said, "I've got it." The person I just had to meet was Elissa Kalver.

The thing that struck me immediately about Elissa was that my fear of small talk had vanished. Elissa doesn't talk small. She dives in. She does the thing I wish I could do in these situations—that is, cut through the pleasantries and go straight to the heart of the matter. The other thing that struck me about Elissa was that she, like me, understood what it was like to live with cancer. I am a leukemia survivor, 19 years in remission, and Elissa is currently living with metastatic breast cancer. We have both used our cancer journeys to create nonprofit organizations that make life easier for cancer patients, survivors, and their loved ones.

Our bond was immediate, but if that rooftop conversation was a dance, Elissa was leading.

Her vitality and sense of urgency were immediately apparent. She didn't just want to talk about our shared bond of disease. She wanted to know how we could work together to help others. This was not a theoretical conversation. Calendars and events were compared on the spot, and I left that night with a new friend and two concrete dates that our organizations would collaborate on to support the cancer community.

In the weeks that followed, I watched from afar as Elissa rappelled down a skyscraper, gave interviews on national television, and hosted an event where women translated their shared cancer experiences into ten-minute standup comedy routines. I'm a pathologically energetic and hardworking person, but Elissa puts me to shame. Her commitment to the cause of living well has inspired me to do more, be better, and think twice about how I choose to spend my days. I wasn't the least bit surprised to find out that Elissa, while juggling motherhood, public speaking engagements, full time philanthropy, and ongoing cancer treatment, had also written a book. The wisdom distilled in *We Got This* is not just a road map for cancer patients, survivors, and the communities that support them. It is a testament to the human spirit and how to live a purpose-filled life.

There is no pretension here. Elissa's gift is not only showing her reader how to thrive in the midst of a calamity, but how to thrive regardless. You don't need to be in crisis to pull wisdom from these pages. You simply need to be a human in search of a better life. I think that's what drew me to Elissa that night in Detroit. Her humanity is always on full display and vibrates with compassion and is completely void of artifice. Her approach to living is pure, intentional, and filled with a desire to wake the world up to all the good that can be drawn from a day. Whether she's rappelling down a skyscraper or hard at work bringing practical relief to people fighting cancer, she is a daily reminder of our ability as humans to create beauty from pain.

Andrew McMahon

Vocalist, pianist, and primary lyricist for Something Corporate and Jack's Mannequin; leukemia thriver; founder of Dear Jack; and author of *Three Pianos: A Memoir*

February 2025

INTRODUCTION

A Message from the Author

My name is Elissa Kalver, and I have stage IV metastatic breast cancer.

I begin my public speaking engagements this way to set the stage. I want to be straightforward about my life with cancer.

When people meet me, they don't assume I have a terminal illness. I'm not bald, and I don't have a family history of cancer. I was thirty-four years old, with an almost one-year-old daughter at home, when I received the phone call that told me I had cancer. After undergoing an ultrasound, mammogram, biopsy, and PET scan, my husband, Eric, and I learned that I had—and still have—HER2-positive metastatic breast cancer. Our doctors told us that this form of cancer can grow and spread fairly rapidly.

They were right.

By the time the disease was fully diagnosed, the cancer had already spread from my breast to my lymph nodes, liver, and lower spine. It eventually spread to parts of my brain as well.

After facing the freezing-cold blast of shock that the diagnosis brought with it, my next thoughts were, *Okay, so what do we do to fight this venomous, unwanted visitor that's been bold enough to invade my body? What do we do to beat it back and kick its ass?*

The answer was simple: *We do everything we can.*

So why am I writing this book? For a bunch of different reasons, all of them pressing, urgent, and, in many ways, life defining.

I'm writing this book to redefine what it means to succeed and to push past the conventional (and often very limited) understanding of what it means to really live life. I want to explain and describe how I stepped into a far more expansive space and a far deeper level of understanding, hoping that my experiences can open up similar paths of growth in your life, if growth is what you're seeking. I'm writing this book to explore what it feels like to actually live every minute of each day, to value and truly experience it.

But here's the thing—cancer shouldn't be a prerequisite for living your best, fullest, most satisfying life. (In fact, that would be pretty awful.)

My goal in writing this book is to share my life experiences and encounters to show how I've come to thrive and live my best life. My hope is that, by sharing my journey, you can find the biggest value in your life—cancer or not.

After getting my diagnosis, I knew that the fight ahead wouldn't be easy, but I also knew it was possible. For me, it meant beginning with my first eight rounds of chemotherapy.

I knew that I would have to summon every ounce of strength within me to fight this fight, and I would do anything and everything to win this long-haul battle. I had a daughter to raise, a husband to love, family and friends to nurture, people to help, and life left to live. My long-term goal was, of course, to live. To beat the cancer. To survive.

My primary short-term goal immediately came into perfect focus: to make it through the eight rounds of chemo.

I learned something important about myself: I was more resilient than I had ever thought possible, more adaptable than I had ever imagined. This is when my definition of "success" began to open up and unfold: My success—both short term and long term—was now suddenly tied to my ability to survive chemo. If I didn't successfully meet the short-term goal of surviving chemo, I wouldn't successfully meet the long-term goal of surviving life. I had no choice but to fight this fight with as much tenacity as I possibly could.

I began to understand something else very important about goal setting: Our goals change and shift based on the situations we face in life. We are constantly adjusting, readjusting, and recalibrating our definition of success; we move the "finish line" to different locations based on our life experiences, which I take as a very good thing because it speaks to the resilience of the human spirit.

In this book I want to take a close look at our resilience and our capacity to live our lives fully, authentically, and with a wide-open heart. I want to share the hard questions that my cancer diagnosis forced me to ask myself: "What am I capable of?" "What matters most to me?" "Am I truly living the fullest and most authentic life I can possibly live?"

Each of us has unique challenges. Everyone is running their own race, with different finish lines built along the way. In each chapter I will share the following message of empowerment: At any point, for any reason, and in whatever fashion you choose, you have the capacity to reposition your finish lines. To pause for a rest and a reset. To change your route, alter your path, and strip away the stuff that's getting in your way.

This doesn't always ensure that you'll *win* the race, but it serves as a reminder that how you choose to run it—which tools you use, which resources you employ, and which direction you take—is a matter of your own personal choice.

I use the finish line metaphor because I also happen to be a distance runner. I'm not an Olympian by any means, but I have run a few marathons, triathlons, and century rides, including a one-hundred-mile bike ride around Lake Tahoe. The parallels I see between living with cancer and running a race are strikingly similar.

When I finished those first eight rounds of chemo, I'd reached a vitally important milestone. I flew across that finish line with the speed and determination of a gold medal sprinter. I'd finished this leg of the race, accomplished my mission, and achieved my goal. When I rang that victory bell at the infusion center (the bell that cancer patients often ring when they've finished their last round of chemo), I rang that damned thing with such force that it broke. I was the *winner* that day, even though I wasn't done with cancer.

This is what we'll explore together: the powerful realization that we have the capacity to expand and redefine what success and victory look like at any point in our lives. How could we *not* be empowered by this knowledge?

The theme that I will keep returning to in this book is that this sense of empowerment belongs to all of us. It belongs to anyone who wants to live life without fear, without regret, and with the absolute knowledge that you are deserving of joy and worthy of its pursuit. This is not just a living-with-cancer principle; this is a living-your-*life* principle, whether you are a cancer thriver or not.

In the spring of 2024, I went on a "cancer trip" with an organization called Project Koru, which uses community and the outdoors as a way to move forward with and beyond cancer. It was a week on a beach in Costa Rica, sharing a house with a dozen amazing cancer thrivers.

Every morning we started with a yoga and journaling session, taking time for ourselves to connect and reflect. We didn't have to reflect on our cancer experience, but for many of us, it was a great space to do that—a safe, welcoming space surrounded by people who got it. On one morning later in the week, I was reflecting on that really difficult period in my life and on the common saying of "living like I was dying"—a phrase that allegedly makes you put things in perspective because time is short, and you have to make every second count. For me, it morphed into a different saying. I didn't want to live like I was dying, as that meant I was limited and that I was only doing things out of fear. I wanted to act out of passion, interest, and purpose. I wanted to live like I'm alive.

I shared at the end of the journaling session, and when I revealed that insight, the group immediately responded. "Oohs" and nods of agreement flew around our little circle. It resonated with everyone. (Some of them even got tattoos of it on the last day of camp!) At one point we all shared the goal of surviving our cancers. But we were all there because we didn't want to just "not die"—we wanted to live.

Today my goals are different simply because my life is different. Those first few rounds of chemo are behind me, and I've been through many treatments since then, but my race is far from over. I will have to aggressively fight this cancer for the rest of my life. I will never *not be* in a fight mode with this disease—at least not until a cure is found, which may not happen in my lifetime. Living with stage IV metastatic breast cancer is a lifelong marathon that I can never stop running. If I stop running, if I stop my treatments or decide to take a rest from this race, the cancer will recur.

My plan—my inexhaustible goal—is to keep running this race with every ounce of energy within me and to do it with joy rather than fear, with positivity rather than pessimism. I am grateful to have this perspective and to have this book as my platform.

To be clear, I am not grateful to have cancer; it sucks. But in a very real way, my diagnosis has given me a mission, a message, and the irrefutable knowledge that I have no time to waste on nonsense or negativity.

If I'm being honest, my diagnosis has also given me a certain level of street cred. Let's face it, I wouldn't even be writing this book if I didn't have cancer. And chances are, if I didn't have cancer, you probably wouldn't be reading this, either. This diagnosis allows me to explore some important themes and principles from a place of total authenticity and raw honesty. It has been a powerful experience to be able to write about life knowing I might die. I'm not being melodramatic; I'm just saying that my cancer has become a *credential* that I did not have before. It has given me a perspective worth sharing . . . so share I will.

My cancer has also been very freeing for me, in a very real sense. I am not romanticizing my illness or sugarcoating it in any way. I'm simply acknowledging—perhaps even celebrating—the fact that I have arrived at a point where I have released all judgments about myself and others, and I don't waste a second worrying about how or if other people judge me. My time is too precious to waste.

I live in a space of pure honesty and, yes, even gratitude. My diagnosis has allowed me to be who I've always been—that same old Elissa—only magnified a thousandfold. I'm grateful that through my work, I am able to shine this bright light into the lives of people (namely, cancer warriors and their supporters) who can really benefit from its warmth and megawattage.

So yes, I can safely say that my "finish line" has now expanded exponentially. When I was first diagnosed, all I wanted to do was survive. To not die. Today I am doing far more than merely surviving. I am thriving. I am living fully because I am worthy of such a pursuit and because I know I am not running this race just for myself but also for the people I love, for the people who love me, for the people I've yet to meet, and for the other cancer warriors whose lives I want to continue to enrich and uplift.

Although this book has a vast audience because its messages can apply to *all* of us, I will direct much of my energy toward my fellow cancer warriors. They are my brothers and sisters; they are the group to whom I have devoted the rest of my life to helping—

not just because I am a member of their "family" but also because bringing comfort, connection, practical resources, and joy is helpful to them. It's deeply rewarding to me as well, simply because I love to help others. It just feels right.

This is another aspect I will celebrate in my book: the grounding and gratifying feeling of being of service to those in need. In my life, it has always been the fuel that propels me. It's just that the cancer has added a jet-fueled intensity to my commitment to helping others.

Reaching out, forming collaborations—with my husband, Eric, always at my side—and providing support and resources to other cancer survivors renew our mission exponentially. It keeps both of us focused, intentional, and on a steady path. (I devote an entire chapter to the importance of people helping people, a driving principle in my life that has never felt as profound as it does today. And for that, I am grateful.)

In fact, my cancer diagnosis led to the creation of my nonprofit, WeGotThis.org, a marketplace and gift registry for cancer patients and their supporters.

Another important reason I'm writing this book is to recognize and celebrate the mission of my nonprofit and to let people know what an amazing, life-enriching resource it has proven to be for those living with cancer.

I decided to start the organization when I was at a particularly difficult point in my treatment. Rather than sulk about my situation, I decided I had to *do* something—to create something that could shine a brighter light into a dark situation. Helping other cancer warriors provides a level of normalcy in my life as well. Talk about silver linings.

The mission statement of WeGotThis.org is "to empower the cancer community to thrive, not just survive, by providing a nonprofit universal gift registry, trusted recommendations, and essential resources—transforming the act of giving and receiving support throughout every cancer experience.

Here I'd like to draw another parallel between the mission statement of my nonprofit and the mission of this book that you are holding right now: In the same way that WeGotThis.org allows cancer thrivers to live their very best lives, I hope this book will uncover ways for you to live yours as well. After all, isn't that what it's all about? Living the very best life we possibly can?

Sure, the choices we make and the paths we take will be different for each of us, simply because we are all unique. Your story is different from my story. If you happen to live with cancer and you're reading these words right now, it's highly unlikely that your cancer is exactly the same as mine. But we're still members of the same club of thrivers—*all* of us, whether we live with cancer or not. We belong to each other.

Within these pages, you will also find—and feel—this collaborative energy because this journey is not just mine alone. It's yours, too.

I've written this book for *everyone*, which, by its very definition, also includes **you**.

I'd also like to add a few gentle disclaimers right up front to help explain my usage of certain words and phrases. When referring to people living with cancer, I sometimes use the terms "patient," "survivor," and "thriver" interchangeably.

I am empathetically aware that everyone identifies differently, and I personally identify myself as a "thriver." You'll see that I will sometimes switch it up, depending on the situation and how I see myself in a particular context. If you have or had cancer yourself, just know that I see you, and I empathize with you. As you read this book, I invite you to swap any of these terms in a way that makes contextual sense to you.

I also use the word "journey" on occasion, and I want to be clear that I know not all cancer patients/survivors/thrivers like this term. I'm not oblivious or ignorant to the dissonance this word can create, but I am a cancer patient, and I choose to use the word because this is what it feels like to me: a journey. If the word makes you bristle, please cut me a break, give me a pass, because I am solely speaking from my experiences. (And if you don't have cancer, you can ignore this paragraph altogether since it's probably not a term you've thought much about in this particular context.)

A final word on verbiage: The last thing I want is for anyone to feel bad. If you read something and think, *Oh man, I've said that before and probably shouldn't have*, it's okay! Let's cut each other some slack. Let's give each other some grace. After all, we're on this "journey" together as a team.

Together, we got this!

CHAPTER ONE

SURVIVING IS NOT ENOUGH

Some Straight-Up Truths

Let's face it, talking about cancer can be extremely uncomfortable and even intimidating. For loved ones and supporters who may not be as intimately familiar with how to have open, honest conversations with cancer patients, the angst and anxiety can be even greater. I want to be candid and up-front about how we talk about cancer, right from the very beginning.

It's important to share some straight-up truths right from the start that might help facilitate communication with cancer thrivers in a way that allows for sensitivity and grace. I share these straight-up truths not to fuss or gripe but to enlighten those who may be unaware of the impact of their words.

Understand that I'm speaking from my personal experience, not on behalf of every person living with cancer. This list is from a place of love and with a little humor in my heart, hoping that you will receive it (and use it!) as a practical, instructive communication tool.

Here is a "quick list" of sayings and sentiments that should be avoided at all costs if you're speaking to someone living with cancer.

Sentiments That Make Me Cringe

The Cringe: "You're so strong. I know you're going to *beat* this!"

There is no cure for stage IV metastatic breast cancer. By the stereotypical definition, that means I can never "beat it." As of now, the best I can do is keep this cancer at bay with aggressive treatment, which I must do until the day I die. This changes my definition of "beating" cancer. I am beating cancer by *living* with it and by living a full and happy life. Please don't tell me I'm going to "beat it."

The Cringe: "My second cousin had breast cancer, too, and we were very close. I understand your journey."

There are almost as many different forms of breast cancer in the world as there are breasts! Cancer is as unique as a fingerprint. Of the hundreds, maybe thousands, of people I know with breast cancer, not one of their cases is exactly like mine. Yes, there are specific types and categories of cancer, but every journey—like every human—is unique and different. I am not a breast. I am not my cancer. I am a human being. I am a human being who happens to have cancer. I love when cancer can connect people through shared empathy. And I know you're speaking from a place of love, but please honor my individual journey because it is uniquely mine—just like your second cousin's was uniquely hers!

The Cringe: "Keep your eye on the prize! You're still *alive!*"

I am certainly grateful to be alive, of course, but my gratitude is far larger and all-encompassing than the mere beating of my heart.

My happiness is not just about avoiding death but also about embracing the fullness of life.

My eye is on the prize of living a balanced, happy, and mission-driven life (such as starting WeGotThis.org, which helps others with cancer live their very best lives). My hopes are pinned not just on waking up alive tomorrow morning but also on living every second of my day as fully as I possibly can. My life is larger than my cancer.

The Cringe: "Keep your chin up. You got this."

While I appreciate the encouragement, when I hear "**You** got this," it dampens my collaborative spirit. I am all about teamwork. I am all about working together to ensure that none of us feels alone or isolated. When you say to me, "You got this," it feels like you are releasing yourself from my team. Certainly, I am the one with the disease, and I am the one going through the treatments, but I have an entire community of supporters behind and around me to remind me that I am never really alone.

Rather than saying "you" got this, why not use the more all-encompassing word "we"? This teamwork concept is exactly what led me to name my nonprofit "We Got This." The "We" is absolutely everything.

Even before I was diagnosed, my cancer had spread from my breast to my lymph nodes, liver, and lower spine. (There were so many tumors on my liver, for instance, that they had difficulty counting them all.) Things took an even more daunting turn when we discovered a recurrence in my left breast and new tumors in my brain.

Here's another straight-up truth: Even though the cancer had spread to other parts of my body, I still just have breast cancer. People often assume (incorrectly) that when it spreads, it changes. I'm not saying that it's impossible for someone to contract multiple types of cancer—it does happen—but more often than not, the original form of cancer simply metastasizes to other parts of the body. I do *not* have liver cancer, brain cancer, or any other type of cancer other than breast.

I want to bring clarity here because it's such a common (and innocent) mistake that deserves correction. Wiping away misconceptions also helps wipe away some of the mystery and melodrama of the disease, which is essential. Cancer is pretty damn dramatic all on its own.

I Choose to Thrive

After recovering from the initial shock of my cancer diagnosis, I went directly into survival mode, into *fight* mode. I did not pass go. I did not collect $200. I went directly to the "boxing ring" to begin the fight of—and for—my life. I put on my gloves, proceeded to my corner of the ring, and surrounded myself with the coaches, trainers, and supporters in my life who would help me fight. Then I went about the business of doing whatever was necessary to battle this bitch called cancer.

Never once did I feel like I was in that ring by myself.

I am (and always have been) constantly surrounded by people who love me, who want the best for me, and who will help me move mountains to keep this disease at bay for as long as possible.

Ultimately, of course, I know that my life belongs to me alone and that when I go in for treatment, this body of mine is the only one receiving that treatment. But it still feels like I have an entire community sitting right by my side, cheering me on and reminding me that I am not alone. They are ready, willing, and able to continue working closely with me, shoulder to shoulder, to help others with cancer lead positive, productive, happy lives.

This close-knit but very far-reaching community, with my husband, Eric, and my daughter, Ellie, firmly rooted at the very center, helps me survive. Equally important, they help me *thrive*. Together, we are firmly bound and directly connected. We are a team. Even though I must navigate the occasional detour and the inevitable bump in the road—don't we all?—my support system is my solid rock, my source of unchanging love in a constantly changing world. We are singular in focus yet amazingly diverse and inclusive.

I will devote the rest of my life to ensuring that those of us within the cancer community (not just the warriors but the supporters, too) experience this same sense of connection, comfort, and belonging.

Our focus? To create, maintain, and nurture a community where everyone with cancer can live with dignity, grace, and happiness. No one among us should have to live with this disease feeling unseen, unheard, or powerless. That's what this community—specifically WeGotThis.org—is all about: coming together to share resources, provide information, and empower each other with the knowledge that we, too, have a voice and a choice in how we live in this world with cancer. We never, ever have to run this race alone.

If there's one thing I've learned on this marathon, it's that

I do not need to endure suffering to prove my resilience.

No one does. This certainly doesn't mean that I won't endure challenging moments along the way—I mean, hardships are a part of life, too—but there must be room for happiness as well. Believe it or not, the two things can coexist.

The simple truth is this: I was in survivor mode precisely when I needed to be. I did what needed to be done to make it through those initial treatments, fully prepared to endure whatever it took to survive, because I was told that if my body couldn't endure those first eight rounds of chemo, I wouldn't have survived at all. There was no choice, really. I *had* to survive those first eight rounds if I wanted to survive at all. Period. My only choice was to fight, to do whatever needed doing to make it through those first eight rounds.

I did make it through. I *survived*. I also realized that even in the darkest times, when it felt like nothing was within my control, I still had the capacity to make decisions about my life and my treatment. I still had the power to communicate those decisions to the people around me, even if they seemed to be at odds with what others considered the "right" course of action moving forward. (More on this later.)

Today I'm still in that figurative boxing ring—for the rest of my life, I'll have to spar, battle, and dance with this disease to keep it from spreading—but my perspective has expanded exponentially, and I now live a life that involves far more than merely surviving. Today, even though I'm still in treatment, I'm still here—whether I'm at home dancing with my husband and our little girl before bed, standing shoulder to shoulder with others in the community raising awareness for WeGotThis.org., or simply sitting by myself, enjoying a quiet moment in the sun.

My will to survive is the reason I am alive today, but I have also willed myself to cherish every hour and minute, every texture and wrinkle, every messy mishap and joyous victory, simply because this is what it means to live life fully and with mindful intention. I have reassigned my priorities: Living a balanced, happy life is just as important to me as fighting this cancer.

While I've never been one to believe in fate, destiny, or divine coincidence, the fact that I once owned a boxing gym is definitely not lost on me. I already *know* how to spar. I know how to fight, to jab, and to duck. I also know how to teach other people these skills. Since sharing knowledge and resources is what I'm all about (and the very reason I started my nonprofit, which we'll explore in upcoming chapters), I'd say this early business venture prepared me very well for the path I am traveling today.

In this moment, I am not only successfully fighting my cancer but also successfully living my life. I am living proof that it is possible to do both things at once. In those dark, early days of my diagnosis, I lived as if I were dying—because it was a necessary and even mandatory way to live at the time. But today I am living like I am alive.

Each and every one us of can lead a full, balanced life, no matter the struggles we face or the setbacks we must endure. It starts (and ends) with making a choice, with assigning specific and intentional value to this thing called the fullness of life, then making the deliberate decision to go after it, no matter what. It starts by giving yourself both the permission and the freedom to strike the balance between the will to survive and the fierce determination to thrive as well. There is space for both.

Don't get me wrong. It is both appropriate and necessary to focus on the vital matter of surviving, especially if you're living with a serious illness or standing in the midst of a messy life situation. I get that. I really do. But sometimes we place so much of our attention on the problem itself that we forget to appreciate the wide-open space of the living world around us and the fact that there's so much more to life than the problem currently engulfing us.

There were times, particularly early in my treatment, when I was so hyperfocused on the medical challenges of getting rid of the cancer (or at least stopping its spread) that I forgot to embrace the other important stuff in my life. I was just a patient who was desperately trying to either lower this number or finish that round or eradicate that tumor—whatever medical challenge was before me became the only challenge I focused on. I became single minded, and sometimes that fixation was necessary. But more often than not, it was a way to avoid thinking about the other things in my life, the things I might lose. What I didn't realize was, by forgetting to embrace that stuff, I'd kind of already lost them. And I didn't want to do that, either.

Today I am still a cancer patient and will remain one for the rest of my life. But because I have made the choice to expand my perspective and open up my life to a wider space, I am much, much more than that: I am a human who happens to have cancer—surviving, thriving, living each and every moment as completely as I absolutely can. This is the way I see it: Surviving is the minimization of thriving. Thriving requires self-love and action. At this moment, on this day, in this space that is my life, I choose to thrive.

Because I love myself enough to want to.

The Beauty of Clarity

The other thing that I want to address early on is *clarity*. I want to share and perhaps even celebrate the way cancer has brought clarity to (and a deeper understanding of) everything around me.

You can probably already tell that I'm a pretty straightforward person. I've always spoken directly from the heart, with clear-eyed honesty and openness, because that's simply the way I am. I've never had the time or the desire to play with the truth, manipulate facts, or speak out of both sides of my mouth—and I *certainly* don't have time for any of that nonsense today.

Although I've always been highly focused and action oriented, and I've always loved this person that is me, my cancer diagnosis has magnified my already-solid sense of self. Today I have less time—*no* time, really—for self-doubt or negative thinking. My diagnosis has amplified my true character and opened a new portal, which gives me both the permission and the power to be authentically, unapologetically *me*.

As crappy as it is to have cancer, the experience of surviving and thriving with this disease has allowed me to explore, on a far deeper level, the best parts of who I really am, which has been both liberating and empowering. Gaining this level of clarity is possible for *all* of us. It is as possible for you as it is for me.

Having cancer is not a prerequisite for living a full life.

No matter what challenges you're facing in your life, my urgent hope is that you understand and embrace the knowledge that you, too, can stand in this place of unapologetic authenticity. You can make the deliberate decision to understand and appreciate the world around you from a wider, more all-encompassing perspective. This choice belongs to all of us.

The thing about clarity, though, at least in my experience, is that it doesn't always come when you want it to come. It comes when you *need* it to come. I was at the lowest point in my life when a new level of clarity arrived and opened my world in unfathomable ways.

After being diagnosed, I entered a clinical trial that profoundly shifted my perspective and made me fully realize the distinction between surviving and thriving. This newly developed sense of clarity changed my entire trajectory, and it probably saved my life.

The drugs I was taking during the trial were working—my tumors had shrunk significantly, for which I was deeply grateful and extraordinarily relieved—but the side effects were wiping me out. After the infusions, I was usually bedridden, with barely a break between treatments. I was also dealing with some pretty severe gastrointestinal issues, muscle aches, and extreme fatigue.

Doing the math on what my future looked like took me to an even darker place: Since I was getting infusions every three weeks, that meant half of my life would be spent feeling miserable in bed, which just wouldn't work for me. Was this my new normal? The constant pain? The never-ending nausea? Being bedridden and so uncomfortable I could barely move? Was this the quality of life I wanted?

This was when I reached a point where the thought of living was beginning to feel too burdensome and the concept of death became strangely comforting. I wasn't suicidal, but the prospect of death was beginning to take on more warmth and appeal; the idea of its arrival no longer felt like a terrifying threat.

As months passed in misery, I questioned whether I was capable of continuing—or if I even *wanted* to. Was it worth enduring such suffering for the sake of survival? I had promised to fight to stay alive, no matter what it took, for my family and friends. But what about me? Was this life still worth living?

Months of antidepressants, various antinausea medications, and some very clear-sighted conversations with my family and my medical team helped bring me to a moment of life-changing clarity: I couldn't continue on this path of misery. The side effects of the drugs I was taking were causing such despair I knew something had to change.

So I made the decision—*we* all did, including my oncologist and the rest of my medical team—to switch treatments. It was risky, but I knew it was the only choice for me. Living in this "fighting mode" could no longer remain an option, and I knew it, suddenly, with clarity and conviction.

So I spoke up! I voiced my feelings and shared my concerns.

My ability to speak up, to stand up, and to take control over the course of my treatment and the direction of my life is what saved me. It also served as a stunning testament to the power of self-advocacy. The support I received from my medical team and my family was the validation I needed to pursue a better quality of life.

As I reflect on those moments—and even as I type these words right now—tears of gratitude and relief flow freely, and I give myself permission to let these tears come because I am deserving of my own gratitude. These tears stem from an authentic place that I honor and respect. I don't see them as a sign of weakness but as a stunning affirmation that I *do* have a voice and a choice. I could choose to stay alive, but instead I choose to thrive.

This choice belongs to all of us, no matter the situations we face in life. My ability to speak up, to stand up, and to express myself from a place of clarity and confidence (combined with the willingness of my medical team to really listen to my concerns and hear my urgent plea) was a testament to the power of choice that I had awakened within me.

I've said this before, but I want to repeat it because this moment of clarity changed everything for me: Choosing to live, to really live, is the true fight against cancer.

The Cancer of Grief

To create a stronger foundational understanding of my relationship with cancer, I must also explore my deepened relationship with grief. There are powerful parallels.

Like cancer, grief itself can spread and metastasize at an alarmingly rapid rate. It can be toxic; its poisonous tentacles can snatch your breath away and reduce the world around you to a dark, dismal, and very, very small place. Like cancer, the toxicity of grief—if left untreated, unchecked, or simply ignored—has the capacity to be lethal. Again, I speak from my own experience.

But grief, like cancer, can also be transformative—like it was for me—because I deliberately placed myself in the right headspace and gave myself the permission to look at my life through a wider prism that certainly includes my diagnosis but is not totally defined by it.

Have you ever dealt with the heaviness of fresh grief? Perhaps you're struggling with the final vestiges of grief after having experienced a loss from long ago. Whether grief has any role in your life today or not, chances are, you're familiar with its sting and its heaviness.

But grief, like cancer, can also be revelatory and eye-opening if you decide to shift its paralyzing heaviness into something that's more positive and palatable in your life. Just as I could not control the arrival of my cancer, I could not control the arrival or source of my grief. Both things arrived suddenly and created huge and messy imbalances. But if you look closely enough, you'll see something other than darkness inside the hidden folds of something as awful as cancer or as stinging as death. What I have found in both things is a measure of control and acceptance. It took me a while, but I have found both.

Several years ago my brother died, and it shook me to my core.

In many ways I am *still* mourning the loss of my only sibling, shocked to be living in a world without him. My big brother's death brought a pain so intense and a grief so razor sharp I could barely breathe.

For the first time in my life, I experienced a loss so sudden and heart-stoppingly severe that I couldn't quite wrap my head around it. But his death also altered me in unexpected ways—it deepened my understanding of life itself.

My brother, Josh, was three years older than me. We grew up in Andover, Massachusetts. The four of us—my parents, my brother, and I—were a close, comfortable family unit. Sure, we had our differences, particularly when my brother and I moved into adulthood, but that's a normal part of growing up and creating our lives.

His death forced me to ask myself some existential questions for the first time in my life: *What am I **doing** here on this earth? Does anything really matter? What is this life I'm living all about?* It woke me up and opened my eyes not just to the wider world around me but also to my place within it and my connection to it.

I don't want to sound too metaphysical here, nor do I want to wrap myself in a cloak of mystery and intrigue, but it's very important that I capture the depth and breadth of the "opening up" that was occurring inside me.

It is my brother's death and my life with cancer—I know this with certainty now—that have deepened my connection to life itself. It's ironic, isn't it? How the loss of a loved one or the sudden prospect of our own death can deepen our connection to the people and principles we hold most dear. Though it sucks that I have cancer and I hate like hell that Josh died, both of these events have changed me in the most fundamental sense, for the better.

Now that I can reflect on it without being blinded by the pain, I see some of the other similarities between my cancer and my grief: Both experiences have heightened my sense of empathy. Both have made me into a more compassionate, consciously empathetic person. This is one reason my drive to help others, particularly those in the cancer community, is as strong as it is—and the very reason I started my nonprofit.

Josh's death opened the door to a deeper understanding about my cancer. I realized that my life is more than just my cancer, just as it is more than my grief. To live a measured and meaningful life requires balance in both these things. Isn't that what thriving is all about? Living life to the fullest, whether that living includes pain, grief, happiness, empathy? That embraces the endless, sometimes-messy spectrum of emotions and experiences?

If my brother were alive today, I know he'd be right here beside me, cheering me on and helping me fight this fight. I would be helping him, too. Though he ultimately died of an accidental drug overdose, I realize now (because cancer has given me this perspective) that he didn't "lose" his battle with addiction at all; he fought it like hell.

In fact, he *won* his long battle with addiction by working as hard as he did to push through his challenges. He persevered. He refused to give up on his life. He was married, owned a home, worked in our family business, and had a baby on the way, though he would never know the joy of discovering that baby was going to be a boy. Today his son is a clone of him in the most endearing ways.

In that same vein, I haven't "lost" my battle with cancer, either. I am living with it every day of my life. I have a loving husband, a beautiful daughter, faithful friends, and a strong non-profit that improves and enriches the lives of other cancer warriors. I have not lost, and my brother didn't lose, either. He won for as long as he could.

The Fact of the Matter

Do I wish my cancer had been detected sooner? You bet I do.

Do I wish I knew what caused my cancer in the first place? Of course.

But if I spent all my time (or even *some* of the time) pining away at what I could have done differently or even wasting five minutes of my precious time wringing my hands over the fact that I have this dumbass disease, it would give me five less minutes to spend reading bedtime stories to my daughter or driving with my husband to Santa Barbara for the perfect breakfast at Bree'osh. I work hard to be present in every moment because each of them is precious, and we will never get them back.

I can't say I haven't wondered why and how this disease chose *my* body to invade, but it did, even though I lived a healthy, active life and had no genetic predisposition to cancer. Even though I exercised regularly, ate the right foods, avoided the "wrong" foods, and took what I thought were responsible, preventive measures, cancer still found me.

Here's the hard truth: There is no guaranteed, fail-safe blockade that totally prevents the disease. Cancer does not discriminate, nor does it give up easily. It's got lots of tricks up its sleeve.

In a very real way, this makes the topic of prevention even more vital, though if you asked me what more I could have done to keep this disease from invading my body, my answer would still be *nothing*. I would not have done anything differently.

There was nothing more I *could* have done. The fact of the matter is that I have cancer. In the same way that I steadfastly refuse to simply survive, I also refuse to beat myself up over whether I could have done something to prevent this unwanted assailant from arriving at my doorstep.

Still, this issue of awareness and prevention is vital and relevant, so let's explore it together in this next chapter.

CHAPTER TWO

PREVENTION

My Pragmatic Approach to Prevention

Even when I had cancer and didn't know I had it (prediagnosis), I never thought that I would actually *get* it.

I had always led a healthy, active lifestyle and was careful about the foods I consumed and the products I used. I was conscientious about avoiding known carcinogens. To the extent that it was realistic, I was intentional and deliberate in my efforts to prevent any encounter or entanglement with cancer.

Prevention was important to me, as it would be to anyone, but I also wanted to live a balanced and joyful life. I'm human. For instance, even though I was aware that plastics were considered toxic and was always careful to avoid them whenever possible, I was certainly not going to toss out every shred of plastic in my home or introduce a radically extreme no-plastics-anywhere policy simply because it wouldn't have been realistic.

As you might be able to tell by now, I place a high priority on creating and curating a comfortable and balanced life. I'm not interested in living under unrealistic constraints or being trapped in an impenetrable bubble.

Whenever it is within my control, I make the conscious effort to live my life fully, passionately, and intentionally. I refuse to live under the dark shadow of fear and the paralysis that it can often create. To me, fear is the opposite of freedom, and life is too precious (and too short) to be weighed down. I owe myself more than that.

The truth is that no matter what preventative measures we practice, whether they're extreme or moderate, it is still impossible to totally eradicate the possibility of getting cancer. Even though I was conscientious in my preventative efforts and had no family history suggesting a higher risk of getting the disease (I have no genetic mutations and am not genetically predisposed), I still got it. Never once did I suspect that cancer would set its sights on me, much less place me at the center of its radar.

But it did.

Shortly after giving birth to my daughter, Ellie, in July 2020, I began to experience some unusual aches and pains, particularly in my feet. I've always enjoyed playing tennis, but I was beginning to notice that my feet would become numb and swollen while I was playing, sometimes so severely I couldn't wear my tennis shoes comfortably.

Because I've always attacked problems (or even potential problems) head-on, I immediately scheduled a visit with my doctor. If there was an issue of any kind, my intention was to cut it off at the pass as quickly as possible—and I'm still proud of myself for taking those first steps so quickly and decisively.

Avoiding procrastination is an important part of practicing responsible prevention.

If something feels off-balance or unaligned in your body, don't ignore it. Get it checked out. *Go after it.* I know this can be scary and unsettling, but gaining clarity on what you're dealing with as early in the game as possible will be helpful, instructive, and possibly even lifesaving in the long run.

Making the decision to pick up the phone and schedule a doctor's visit is totally within your control. In fact, the decision *belongs* to you. Be your own conscientious advocate, even if it's scary (which it often is).

All my initial blood tests and screenings came back normal, which gave me a measure of comfort, but it still felt like something was off. I was still extremely fatigued, and the aches and pains persisted. I went back to my primary care doctor, to my gynecologist, and even to a rheumatologist, who investigated whether I might be experiencing an autoimmune disorder. Still, nothing disturbing or conclusive, *but I still pushed.* I couldn't let it go because I knew it was something; I just didn't know what that "something" was.

It's important to emphasize here that at no point during this early trajectory did I entertain the possibility that this could be cancer. It never so much as crossed my mind. I now realize, as I reflect on them, that a small part of me was actually grateful that I didn't know yet simply because it made the journey less stressful. I was grateful to live in ignorant bliss, at least for a little while, even though this bliss would soon transform into mind-numbing shock.

One morning, while getting dressed for work, my husband, Eric, found a lump in my breast. The fact that he happened to be—let's see how I can put this—"copping a feel" when he made the actual discovery is proof, in my mind, that there's a silver lining in every dark cloud, right? (I mean, if bad news must be revealed, why not at least have it revealed in the context of an intimate moment?)

Even with the discovery of the lump, though, I wasn't totally convinced it was cancer. I thought it might be related to breast-feeding Ellie—a clogged milk duct or cyst, for instance—even though I hadn't breastfed for about ten months. Clogged duct? Perhaps. But cancer wasn't even on the table, and it wasn't that I was in *denial* about having the disease; I simply didn't think I had it.

When Bright Lights Give Way to Darkness

Once the lump was discovered, things moved pretty quickly. More targeted testing began in earnest at that point, including an ultrasound, a mammogram, and a biopsy. But it was the PET scan (positron-emission tomography, an imaging test used to find tumors and identify a variety of diseases) that revealed my diagnosis: HER2-positive metastatic breast cancer.

Two things from when Eric and I sat together in the surgeon's darkened office that day, as she brought the images onto the screen, will be forever etched into my memory.

The first was what actually showed up on the screen. In a PET scan image, the areas that are cancerous will be revealed by the presence of lights. What I remember, as Eric and I looked at the screen, is the presence of light *everywhere*, which indicated, of course, that the cancer had already spread to different parts of my body.

Never in my life had the presence of so much light created so much darkness.

Lights in my left breast. In my armpit. In my lymph nodes. My lower spine. And my liver was on fire—an angry, seething *wildfire* of lights, bright enough to illuminate the darkened office. Eric and I both sat, staring, stunned.

Eric's expression is the other image I'll always remember—frozen. He seemed completely suspended in time and space as the magnitude of what he was seeing slammed into him.

When he began hyperventilating, the nurse gave him a brown paper bag to breathe into. The bag was already there, kept close at hand for moments exactly like this. It felt uncomfortably impersonal for what we were going through. But for them—the surgeon, the nurses, the doctors—news like this, a reaction like Eric's, were entirely routine. Probably mundane. Every day. Though they just wanted to help, to keep Eric from further hyperventilating, it felt like a formulaic, cookie-cutter response to his deeply human emotion, which didn't feel right at all.

They handed us a single sheet of paper with a list of resources and organizations we could contact, if we chose to, that might be helpful as we started down this arduous path.

While I realize that a sincere effort was being made to share vital information and resources, the way it was done left more than a little to be desired. There was just *something* about that single sheet of paper being placed into our hands so mechanically that made me squirm.

Even in the middle of my own shock, I made a mental note to myself that if I were ever in a position to help others with cancer, I would do it with compassion, tenderness, and the awareness that cancer patients are human, too. Those of us who live with this disease need to feel like we're being seen and heard. We need to be treated like the humans that we are. My shock that day was real, as was my need for compassion and tenderness. Certainly medical professionals have a job to do, and they are not therapists, comforters, or friends, but I still believe that there is always room for compassion, dignity, and respect. I don't ever want someone's personal experience or their life to become "cookie cutter" to me. If I were ever in a position to provide other cancer patients with information and resources, I'd do my best to offer them with as much compassion, love, and humanity as possible.

Those few moments in the surgeon's office that day ended up being of great value as we began creating our nonprofit. In everything that we do for and with cancer thrivers and their supporters, we do it with empathy, sensitivity, and respect.

We are human first, patients second.

Sitting there together that day, although both of us were overwhelmed, *I found my voice.* With Eric hyperventilating beside me and the bright lights of my cancer lighting up the darkened room, I found my voice. In fact, I think it was Eric's intense reaction that forced me into a calmer state. I simply began asking the surgeon questions: "What does stage IV metastatic breast cancer **mean** exactly?" "Am I receiving, in this moment, the prognosis that I only have a few more months to live?" "How are we to interpret the presence of all these lights?" "What has to happen next?" I needed to find the right way to ask the real question, the scary question:

"Am I dying?"

All those lights had suddenly brought everything into focus. They not only illuminated the areas where cancer was present but also brought intense clarity: Cancer was now a part of our reality. We snapped ourselves out of our initial paralysis to take whatever action was necessary, whatever next steps were needed to be taken. We needed to be clear sighted, resourceful, and confident. My life literally depended on it.

Becoming "nicely aggressive" in those early days of my diagnosis was vital. I was aggressive about getting additional tests scheduled. I was pleasantly persistent about getting in to see the right doctors and tenacious about making sure I got seen in a timely manner, as there was no time to lose and even less to waste. After his initial panic, Eric swiftly and assuredly slipped into his role as advocate, supporter, partner, and protector—the role he still plays so beautifully in my life today.

Another lesson I learned? If you are on a cancer journey—or any journey that requires swift, decisive action to complete—learn to become *nicely aggressive*. Ascertain the information and resources that will be most helpful to you as quickly and efficiently as possible, and ask for what you need without preamble or apology.

This is also a time to surround yourself with advocates who can act on your behalf, who can amplify and communicate your needs to others, and who can bring balance and normalcy into your life when it feels like so much around you is crumbling. Look for these people. Create collaborative, meaningful partnerships with them; they are your advocates.

While Eric is certainly my fiercest advocate, there are others in my life whose knowledge and expertise also help steer the course of my trajectory. Don't be shy about seeking these people out. Be resourceful. If you're normally shy and hesitant, you'll need to throw those characteristics overboard for a little while—at least until you can steer your ship back on course. If you're facing a serious downturn in your life, if the waters around you are choppy and the waves are high, do not be discouraged. You are not alone. People in your life who can act as lifesavers and beacons exist. Find them.

Immediately after receiving my diagnosis, I shared the news with two very important people in my life: my stepfather, Dr. Leslie Selbovitz, former chief medical officer of Newton-Wellesley Hospital with over five decades of experience as a distinguished internist, and Eric's uncle, Dr. Charles Elboim, a highly respected breast surgeon with over fifty years of experience. Both of these brilliant doctors worked with me to develop a list of highly specific questions to ask my own doctors moving forward.

If you've been newly diagnosed, cast a wide net and make a list of people and resources that can support you on this journey. You do not need to travel this road alone, but you must maintain clarity of mind, allowing you to see your situation clearly, without the heavy weight of fear or the paralyzing power of panic and anxiety holding you down. It's not about finding a way to "smile through it." There's enough toxic positivity in the world. This is about finding what and who you need to make it through.

Above all, as I mentioned earlier, *be your own advocate*—and advocate for the people in your life. Particularly in the initial stages of dealing with my diagnosis, in addition to seeking advice and counsel from those I knew could help, I also became a huge advocate for myself.

I tracked down surgeons. I demanded (politely) that appointments be scheduled. When doctors didn't call back, I called them again, undaunted and fully determined to get the information I needed, even if it was just to schedule an appointment. I demanded (politely) the necessary attention from the people who mattered, and I required (pleasantly) that everyone on my care team keep me closely in the loop. I refused to let decisions be made without me, particularly since those decisions were being made on my behalf.

How do I weave all these threads together in a way that pulls the topic of prevention into a single fabric? By emphasizing how important it was (and is) for me, at all times, to be persistent, unapologetically vocal, and constantly aware of what's going on around me, not only as I travel this cancer journey but also as I live my life in general. Awareness is a vital component of prevention; the two things are inextricably linked.

In that same vein, playing an intentionally proactive role in our own health, even in a general sense, is a critical part of preventative care. Even though I have cancer, I am proud of the preventative steps I took to avoid it. I refuse to beat myself up about the fact that, despite my best preventative measures, I ended up getting it anyway. I will not live in regret; regret is an emotion that does not belong to me. I have no room for it in my life. Cancer is part of my life, yes, but it is not the *only* part—and I am confident that there was nothing else I could have done to prevent its arrival.

Don't Let People Get Inside Your Head

Once it was visibly clear that I was living with cancer—the beanie on my head, my baldness when I was undergoing chemo—the unsolicited advice from others came flying at me in a constant torrent.

As it concerns prevention, almost everyone has a sentiment or two to share. So here are a few more cringeworthy moments, those times when things were said that should have been left unsaid. Use them as a guide for how to communicate with a cancer thriver—and how *not* to.

A Few More Sentiments That Make Me Cringe

The Cringe: "Excuse me for asking, but I see you don't have hair. Are you in chemo? Can I ask if you're on any type of special diet?"

In the past, whenever anyone asked me "the diet" question, I'd answer it fully . . . until it dawned on me that I don't *have* to answer someone's question just because they ask it!

Today, rather than launching into a detailed response, I counter the question with a question, such as "Why do you ask?" This allows me to get to the true motive of why the person is asking the question in the first place, and more often than not, they're asking because they have a particular diet that they're preparing to share. *No, thank you.*

To those who don't live with cancer, remember that every person who does (live with cancer, that is) is unique. The diet or food preference that works for one person will not automatically work for another. We are humans, not automatons. Please don't oversimplify my cancer by approaching me with a one-size-fits-all solution. Think through your intention before asking an insensitive or unfeeling question. Also, please don't make judgments about the state of my medical condition based on the clothing I wear. I don't do that to you; don't do it to me.

Case in point: At the end of a very long, difficult day some time ago, I decided to treat myself to a frozen yogurt. The employee behind the counter, noticing I was wearing a beanie and was obviously bald underneath, told me I should be drinking dandelion tea, *not* eating frozen yogurt! Normally, I would have said something like, "Look, lady, I'm only trying to find a friggin' sliver of happiness by having this frozen yogurt after a pretty crappy day, so grant me that simple peace, if you don't mind."

But even in anger, there is space for grace. Because I happened to be in a fairly magnanimous mood, I only said something like, "Thanks for that. I'll take it under advisement," then I walked out of the shop, enjoyed every spoonful of my yogurt, and steadfastly refused to let her get inside my head.

There is so much I cannot control as I navigate this cancer journey, but deciding who gets inside my head is something over which I have ultimate control.

The Cringe: "Don't you feel fortunate that breast cancer is one of the most common forms and the easiest to treat?"

Not too long ago, I was preparing to play tennis with someone I'd never met. The woman who'd arranged the match introduced me to my opponent, and during the introduction, she mentioned the fact that I was battling breast cancer, to which my future opponent responded, "Oh well, at least it's the *good* kind of cancer."

Without missing a beat, I answered, "Oh, I didn't realize that terminal cancer, which is what I have, is the 'good' kind.'"

It was a knee-jerk reaction, I know, and more than a little snarky, but it was appropriate and fitting. Statements like hers place a needless burden on those of us living with cancer. Why must I constantly weigh the challenge of whether to put someone in their place? I will not exert my valuable energy trying to figure out how to respond to questions like these. Even if they're coming from a place of love, they're also coming from a place of ignorance, and I deserve more respect than that.

My cancer doesn't require me to be gracious and forgiving of other people's callous inconsideration. Sometimes, maybe. But I will always reserve the right to snap back.

The bright side of this story—and there's always a bright side—is that by the end of the match, we were getting along just fine. I continued speaking with her, and our conversation expanded far beyond cancer.

Oh, and I also wiped the court with her.

The Cringe: Filling out medical history forms.

The simple act of filling out a medical history form isn't *always* cringeworthy, of course, but the questions on those forms certainly give me moments of pause and even reflection, if only because they serve as simple reminders that my cancer will forever be a part of my medical history. Even if you're a warrior whose cancer has gone into remission, it will always be a part of your history.

I've always been drawn to the saying, "It takes longer to recover from cancer than it does to treat cancer." It's a simple reminder that cancer is a lifelong journey. Having cancer automatically places you in a club that you didn't ask to join, yet you're a member for life. Sure, there are some members of this club who are gracious and wonderful, but if given the choice, I'd just as soon decline the membership!

Whenever I'm required to complete a medical history form and I arrive at the section where they ask how many children I have, I always write "one," but immediately thereafter comes the question of how many times I have been pregnant. To that question I must always answer "two" because I had a miscarriage before Ellie was born.

That, too, is not only a part of my medical history but also an important part of my *life*, and it will remain with me always. I'm not saying that I don't want to remember it; I'm saying that when I *do* remember it, I definitely still feel the sharp tug on my heart.

These are impactful moments that stay with us forever. They have a place within our DNA. Our past is our present in a very real way. If you search your medical history, and I'm sure you'll come across something that stirs those same emotions and pulls those same heartstrings.

Facts, Stats, and Other Voices on the Topic of Prevention

Since an important part of preventing cancer is increasing our awareness of the disease, I want to conclude this chapter by sharing some objective, empirical information and by amplifying the voice of a noted authority on the topic. We fight cancer with information, not with misinformation and fear. To the extent that we can prevent it, we prevent it with purpose, passion, and intention.

Facts and Figures About Metastatic Breast Cancer
(Source: METAvivor: Metastatic Breast Cancer Research, Support and Awareness)

- 115 individuals die each day from metastatic breast cancer in the United States.

- 30 percent of all breast cancer patients will metastasize.
- Only 2–5 percent of funds raised for breast cancer research is focused on research for the already metastasized patient.

A Voice of Reason and Authority

Dr. Eleonora Teplinsky, head of breast and gynecologic medical oncology at Valley Health System in New Jersey, speaks passionately about metastatic breast cancer.

She is not only a nationally recognized authority figure but also has become a trusted friend with whom I have collaborated with.

When I was a guest on her podcast, she reflects on a few of the challenges faced by patients with metastatic breast cancer while also balancing her words with optimism and hope.

At some point the treatment may stop working. The cancer cells become resistant and develop ways to outsmart the therapy, so we have to pivot to a different therapy. Luckily, there have been incredible advances over the last few years that are allowing people to live longer, and there are new therapies. When one stops working, we have treatment options.

Patients with metastatic breast cancer are often on prolonged therapies or even lifelong therapy, so *quality of life* becomes of utmost importance when we balance the medications and their side effects with the patients' day-to-day.

Never Be Careless with Cancer

As we bring this chapter on prevention to a close, I want to return to the notion that it is both vital and necessary to take preventative measures to keep cancer as far away as possible. I never want to be cavalier or careless about what I say or write about the subject of prevention.

Yes, I happen to have stage IV metastatic breast cancer, which is "terminal" by its very definition because 100 percent of all cases eventually end in death. There is no cure. But this sobering statistic doesn't mean I think I will die tomorrow, nor does it absolve myself of the responsibility to share the urgent message that taking preventative measures is both our right and our responsibility.

Our ability to make intelligent choices and equip ourselves with the necessary information and resources to live full, meaningful lives—whether we are living with cancer or supporting someone who is—belongs to each and every one of us.

For the rest of my life, I am committed to helping those who are on this journey.

I want us to not just survive but also thrive.

I want us to stand strong in the knowledge that our voices are being heard and that we can use them to obtain the things we need to make this journey more comfortable, more palatable, and more joyous. In fact, being able to decide on and obtain the things that made me comfortable during those first difficult rounds of chemo is what turned my life around—and the reason I started WeGotThis.org.

Helping others, particularly cancer thrivers and their supporters, is what gives direction and definition to my world and my life, and it happens to be the topic of the next chapter.

CHAPTER THREE

PEOPLE HELPING PEOPLE

Better Together

I've been driven by this concept of "better together" for as long as I can remember, long before my diagnosis. It's a principle I put into practice every single day, and it brings purpose, balance, and happiness to my life. My cancer only crystallized the concept and magnified its intensity. If there's a problem that needs to be solved or a gap that needs to be filled, we are *better together* than we are isolated and apart. I am not an island, and neither are you.

I've always enjoyed working on teams, moving in tandem with others, and coming up with creative, collaborative solutions to problems in ways that benefit *everyone* involved. In fact, let me lay claim to my collaborative energy because *it is certainly one of my superpowers.*

Throughout my childhood and early adulthood, for example, I always enjoyed moving and playing within groups, not just because it was more interesting to me but also because I found it more fun.

In high school I played competitive field hockey, and I was pretty damn good at it. As the captain of the team, it was my responsibility to lead and coordinate, sure, but I was also the one helping my teammates' strengths shine. I was energized by my teammates, and we became masterful at playing off one another, building one another up so that we all became stronger. (Isn't that what teamwork is all about?)

I was eventually recruited to play in college and brought on as the starting goalie. Playing in Europe and earning national gold medals was an adventure, but the most enduring reward from that time is the productive, meaningful relationships with my former teammates that I still enjoy to this very day.

In fact, let's scratch the word *former teammates* and use *current teammates* instead because many of them still contribute their energy, time, financial resources, and talents to the task of raising awareness about my nonprofit.

That's how I know we're better together. Even though we're no longer running on the same field, we continue to share a common goal. We still know how to play (and work) as a team to this very day, is proof that our collective energy never really dissipated at all. If anything, it increased. When people come together to help other people, they become larger than their own individual pursuits.

Obviously, I still have singular interests and solitary pursuits in my life, but it's the collective teamwork dynamic that excites and energizes me most. This notion of "we" and "us" working together for the greater good not only wakes me up; it also *lifts* me up! When I am working side by side with people whose mission is to help others, it feels like a gust of wind is lifting us up beyond our own individual circumstances and carrying us together toward that common goal.

Another truth I love about people helping people is that when we come together to close a gap, address a need, or solve a problem, the challenges and adversity we face in our daily lives seem to reconfigure themselves. They still exist, of course, but they become more manageable. Less pervasive. Just a little easier to handle.

I don't mean to imply that our issues magically disappear or that the wrinkles in our lives are suddenly smoothed out with the single swoop of a magic wand. But when we involve ourselves in collective causes and team-related activities that make our lives just a little easier and happier, we are giving ourselves permission to look—and to live—beyond the confines of our own adversity.

This concept of "better together" embraces *all* of us. It's not confined to one group, one goal, or one cause. We are human beings who live together in the world, not apart. It takes all of us (not just some of us) to reinforce, solidify, and *activate* this concept.

For me, the act of helping those in the cancer community lead meaningful, balanced, and empowered lives is as important as fighting cancer itself.

I've already described how, when I was first diagnosed, my first thought was, *What do I have to do to fight this thing? Whatever it is, I'll do it.* At the time it was a necessary mental space for me to stand in. During those first few weeks and months after my diagnosis, I was more focused on what I needed to do to *not die* than on what I needed to do to live. There is a difference.

Looking back at those days, I see it with clarity now.

I was scared of dying.

I was scared of leaving my infant daughter without a mother, my husband without a wife and partner, and my family and friends without my loving, living presence.

I was scared of what it would look like to "lose" this fight with cancer.

But as I have traveled this cancer trajectory, I have evolved into a new space.

I am no longer afraid of dying. I am afraid of not living.

When I work in such close tandem with the organizations and volunteers to help others in the cancer community feel empowered and in control, I am living my very best life.

So yes, cancer still sucks, but the silver lining (and as I've written before, there's *always* a silver lining) is that by helping others who live with this disease, I no longer give my own fear the power it once had over my life.

I cannot control the fact that cancer has decided to inhabit my body, but I can exercise complete control over how I choose to live my life and navigate each and every moment. This is the very reason that led me to start WeGotThis.org.

Even though our goal is singular and narrowly focused in its intent—to build a community through giving and receiving that helps cancer thrivers and their supporters live their very best lives—our reach and impact are anything but narrow. The organization is inclusive, fast growing, and hard charging. When people help people—whether it's creating a nonprofit to help cancer thrivers, or building a new community center in your neighborhood, or developing a volunteer outreach program at your job, or even doing a day of service with your company or with some friends—it's a reminder that

life itself is a team sport.

Cancer is a team sport, too.

It Feels Good to Do Good

The intentional act of building strong relationships is not a novel concept by any means. In business it's done every day. Creating mutually beneficial alliances is strategic and wise. It facilitates growth. It ensures stability. It expands your potential client base and lays the groundwork for future development.

But in the business world, the notion that "everyone wins when everyone wins" has its limits. As soon as those balance sheets become, well, a bit unbalanced, or as soon as one party feels like they have reached a point of diminishing returns, then priorities and strategies seem to shift. Adjustments are made. Corrections designed to slow the losses and revive the gains are put into place. When the balance shifts and one party ends up receiving less than the other, the partnership, generally speaking, is either restructured or dissolved. This is when the "people helping people" principle can often lose its allure—when one party simply isn't receiving as much "help" (or as healthy a return on their investment) as the other. This is when corrective steps are taken and the playing field is leveled to ensure more equitable distribution. This is neither bad nor good. It's business.

For me, though, the act of creating collaborative relationships has always been done with a purpose in mind: to bring about a greater good.

As a former financial advisor, I found it extremely gratifying to create partnerships and work cooperatively with others to help them meet their goals. This meant helping companies set up their 401(k) plans and educating the employees on how to enroll in them—a sometimes daunting task, especially since many of these people were just taking their first steps into the world of personal finance.

I actually enjoyed advising people on how best to build for their future, and I always spent as much time as was necessary to make sure they understood the intricacies and implications of everything before them. After all, these were important, life-defining decisions.

It wasn't unusual for me to spend an entire day with the employees who needed guidance and advice on how best to get their plans started—and I still think it was time well spent.

I'd take on as many plans as I possibly could, of any size, including small start-ups and new plans with very few assets. Before I knew it, I'd brought in more 401(k) plans than anyone else in the company (not in assets but in quantity)—and this was only during my first year!

I spent so much time with each of them because they *needed* it. They had important questions that needed answering and intricate, complex financial options that needed exploring, so it was vital that I took the time to thoroughly address all their inquiries, even when those inquiries weren't always directly related to their 401(k)s. I felt like they needed and deserved my attention and expertise, and I felt fortunate to be able to offer it. Helping them navigate this difficult terrain was invaluable to them and meaningful to me.

As a result of these close collaborations, trusting relationships were developed and nurtured over time. People genuinely appreciated the care and attention I gave them when they were new to personal finance and had important "next steps" to take but didn't quite know how. (Many of these people would become valued clients later on and friends as well. Having played even a small role in their growth was and is extremely gratifying.)

I also worked with established, high-net-worth clients and plans. I gave the same time and attention to those who were new to saving as I did to those who already had millions in the bank. I was never shortsighted, and I knew that putting in the work would always make its way back around.

I never focused on how much I made on each individual client or meeting. I zoomed out and looked at the big picture and viewed my clients as *teammates*. I was on their team to help them reach their goals and objectives, and they were on my team to help keep my business growing through either their own accounts, referrals, or both.

I happen to be a member of the cancer community who has figured out, with the help of a growing group of others, how to bring meaning, purpose, and a sense of connection to others living with the disease. I'm uniquely suited to provide this service. If cancer is my cred, then I'm okay with that.

As much as having cancer sucks, I consider myself fortunate to understand the unique needs and sensitivities that cancer thrivers face each and every day. I understand the gaps that need to be filled because I have come face-to-face with them in my life. I have always considered myself lucky to have the collaborative skills, the get-it-done mindset, and the burning desire to bring people together in a way that makes their lives better.

Everyone has experienced the discomfort of coming face-to-face with something that's painful or perplexing and not knowing which way to turn. We know these are the moments when we need each other the most!

I remember what it was like as a young adult to face complex financial decisions that were difficult to grasp but that I knew would have a huge impact on my life moving forward. I remember that sense of confusion, anxiety, and even helplessness, which is why it was important to offer my own skills and expertise to those who'd found themselves at a similar intersection.

When it comes to helping others—at least for me—there is no "optimum time." There is no profit-driven window of opportunity that opens and closes at a particular moment. Helping people is helping people. Period. I will spend the rest of my life devoted to this very task. If you asked me why this passion to help others seems to be embedded in my DNA, I'd probably lead you back to four simple words that distill the answer down to its barest essence:

Because it feels good.

The Toxicity of Tunnel Vision

In all my outreach efforts, I try to view the world through the widest lens I possibly can. I'm intentional and deliberate about keeping my focus expansive rather than narrow and myopic. Tunnel vision is toxic. While blinders have their purpose, wearing them in all situations is not only counterproductive but also dangerous. The trouble is, we don't even realize we're wearing them until we take them off, then suddenly—voilà—we are able to view the world through a wider prism.

Living with cancer has expanded my perspective in ways that I never imagined. I have learned to live in the richness of every single moment. Whether the moment is painful or pleasurable, I have learned to cherish it because it belongs to me. I do not have a minute to spare.

None of us do.

Here's the thing about tunnel vision, particularly as it relates to the "people helping people" principle: If we allow ourselves to become unnecessarily selective (translated: narrow minded) about how we choose to help others, we're not going to be able to help others. It's as simple as that.

As always, I'll use myself as an example.

Some time ago I was approached by an organization I'd worked with in the past. They were beginning to plan their annual benefit, and a board member had reached out to express interest in the possibility of naming WeGotThis.org as the beneficiary! I was both humbled and honored to even be considered, and I promptly sent them the background information they had requested.

About a week later, I received a call saying they were very sorry, but after reviewing the information I'd sent, it seemed that we were not the "right fit" after all. They were looking for an organization to give money to that would simply buy wigs for cancer patients. In other words they wanted to help that element of cancer treatment *they* identified as the most relevant and important, without really focusing on the bigger picture that considered cancer patients' individual preferences and specific needs.

Don't get me wrong. Plenty of patients want wigs, but there's just as many who don't. I like to be inclusive of those who don't choose this option or who may want *other* things to make them happy and comfortable during treatment.

When I probed a little more and asked for a more lucid explanation, the response I received sounded something like this—and I'm placing this in italics instead of presenting it as a direct quote because I'm paraphrasing here:

> *We knew that your organization helped people with cancer, which drew us to you in the first place, but we thought you made wigs and other products. We were under the impression that you manufactured cancer-related gifts and items rather than just existing as a platform. We're very sorry, but we've decided to continue our search.*

This is how I *wanted* to respond but didn't:

No, we don't make wigs. We don't have a "cancer stuff"
warehouse tucked away somewhere with chemo blankets,
baskets of lotions, and other cancer-related products mov-
ing swiftly along on assembly lines, getting prepackaged in
pretty boxes and delivered to the masses. We're a platform.
We're a marketplace and gift registry that allows patients
and their supporters the ability to choose the specific things
they want and need in their lives to make their experience
with cancer easier and more comfortable.

The lesson here is that when we are evaluating how best to help others, we should do everything we can to avoid falling down that slippery slope of selective judgment. We must force ourselves to expand our narrow definition of "help" so that it evolves into a principle—and a practice—that is inclusive, not exclusive. If we don't, we're not helping. Frankly, we're just choosing what makes *us* feel best rather than the person in need. The only person who gets to dictate what they need is the one experiencing cancer. When we think we know what that is—whether because we know someone else with cancer, have had cancer ourselves, or have seen a lot of episodes of *Grey's Anatomy*—we're not really listening and definitely not helping.

I hope this example, as unpleasant as it is, brings relevance and depth to this chapter—namely, that if we're too narrow minded about how we're helping people, we're not going to be able to *actually* help them. It's a piece of wisdom deserving of reflection.

Since WeGotThis.org is a cancer gift registry and I am its founder, I receive texts and emails all the time from people asking for advice on what they should get for their friends living with the disease. I certainly understand (and am grateful for) their desire to give not only with intention but also with *attention*.

But here's the thing: If I responded to each and every message individually, I'd only be able to help the precise number of people to whom I responded. That relatively small number of people would be the only ones who would benefit.

But if I took a more expansive approach and figured out a way to greet these inquiries with an even wider embrace, I could widen my "help circle" exponentially!

So that was what I did.

I took a step back and decided, after a bit of creative collaboration with my team, to create an *entire resource directory* on our website to address these kinds of questions. This way a larger number of people benefit, particularly since many of them are probably grappling with some of these same questions about gift giving!

I still try to answer as many individual inquiries as I can, of course, but in directing those inquiries to our resource directory, I'm freed up to do other essential work within the organization that brings value and benefit to the greatest number of people possible. In this way the help we provide is inclusive and far more impactful.

The other lesson—closely related but beautifully distinct—is so simple: When it comes to people helping people, *the greater good comes first.*

I have committed my life to bringing the greatest good to the largest number of people in the cancer community as I possibly can, and there is nothing that will stand in my way. Not even cancer.

CHAPTER FOUR

WE GOT THIS

From Darkness to Light

You could say it was born in the bedroom.

The idea of creating a nonprofit actually came to me in our spare bedroom.

I'd just finished my fifth round of chemo and was feeling weak, disheartened, isolated (it was also the middle of COVID-19), and very, very sorry for myself. I was sick. I was tired. Yes, I was sick and tired of feeling sick and tired. Without a doubt, it was one of the darkest periods in my life.

I would never have guessed that those dark, destabilizing moments that day would eventually transform into the brightest light I've ever known. There's no way in the world that I could have predicted it.

But that was what happened.

I was not only sick from the chemo, but I was also feeling more disconnected from myself than I ever had before. Reflecting on it now, I realize I was also grieving the cancer itself and how it was transforming my life. I was grieving its unwelcome arrival and the havoc it created, as well the things that I'd lost (or thought I'd lost) because I now had this new beast demanding attention.

I remember thinking, *There's **got** to be another way to feel other than this. If this is my "new normal," then I'm not sure I'm up for this. I know I promised myself to fight to stay alive for my family and for my friends. But what about me? Do I really want to spend the rest of my life **fighting** for my life instead of simply living it?*

I wasn't thinking of actively, intentionally ending my life. I'd just reached a point where the thought of living felt too burdensome, and the concept of death—of not going through all this—was beginning to feel oddly comforting.

I asked myself this question: "Am I ready to give up?"

Luckily, my answer was loud and clear: "Oh, hell no. I'm not going out like this. Fuck cancer."

If I was going to exert any measure of control over the way my life was unfolding, this was the moment. I couldn't control the fact that I had cancer, but I *could* control how I was going to live with this impostor that had invaded my body and my quality of life. I could control the life I was going to curate for myself.

It also hit me, full blast, that it was totally within my power to help other cancer warriors on their journey—those I knew, those I didn't know, those I would one day meet, and even those I might never meet. In our spare bedroom that day, through the scorched earth of my own depression and desperation, the concept of WeGotThis.org rose straight up from the ashes.

The first person I turned to was my husband, Eric, my closest confidant, my best friend, and the person I trust the most in this entire world.

When I told him I was thinking about starting a nonprofit for cancer thrivers, he responded with both an answer and a question: "Of course you are! How could you *not?*"

From that very first moment, and every moment since, Eric has been my fiercest collaborator. We are passionate and intentional in our efforts to raise awareness about (and support for) WeGotThis.org, and to ensure that the organization influences as many lives as possible.

His immediate and unconditional support added wind to my sails and helped solidify, in my mind, that this was something that needed to be done, not just because I wanted to do it but because it would create a greater good within the community.

And that *I was the one to do it.*

Today Eric's passion and presence add focus and fuel to our collective journey. We share the same vision and passion for this organization and for life in general. I couldn't do this without him. The fact that he is a professional musician and an award-winning music supervisor magnifies our ability to bring those in the music industry directly into our orbit as well. *Everyone* wants to help. To contribute. To be a part of a collaboration that helps cancer thrivers live happy, meaningful lives.

Eric's initial reaction of unconditional support was not only gratifying but also energizing; it spurred me on and lifted me up. In fact, most of the people in my close circle of trusted friends, family, and colleagues were supportive of the idea when I first told them. But I also received words of caution and concern from those who were worried that such an ambitious endeavor might be "too much" for me. They told me that I should be "focusing on my treatment" instead of starting a nonprofit. That I should be "taking it easy" rather than charging full speed ahead with a new project that would obviously require an inordinate amount of my time and energy. That I should "conserve my energy" to fight my own cancer instead of focusing on the larger community.

While I realized, even then, that their concerns were coming from a place of love, I hated hearing it. Frustration, anxiety, and even resentment started to build within me.

"You should be conserving your energy" was exactly what I *didn't* need to hear! What energy? I hadn't had any, and "saving" the little I did have for treatment alone was draining my spirit. With this idea, my flagging energy was finally revived by the thought of helping others in the cancer community.

I was beginning to feel mission driven and purposeful again. I didn't need words of warning, even if they were coming from places of love and genuine concern. What I *did* need was to give myself permission to go after the things that would bring meaning, direction, and happiness to my life.

We all deserve as much. We all deserve the chance to go after the things that bring sustenance and balance to our lives. We deserve to be fearless and unapologetic in our pursuit, even if we happen to have cancer. We deserve to go after the big goals, even (perhaps especially) during the toughest of times.

When I reached out to my therapist to share my idea, along with the frustration, resentment, and anxiety I was experiencing from all the warnings I was receiving from others, she simply said, "Elissa, you *deserve* to start something that makes you feel happy and fulfilled."

Her words not only stuck with me; they also propelled me forward.

We all deserve to do the things that make us feel happy and fulfilled, even if others have a different idea of what our happiness should look like.

If there is something that's stirring inside you—a plan, a dream, an idea, or the *beginnings* of a plan, a dream, or an idea—that not everyone in your life will embrace, trust and love yourself enough to take the leap anyway. If that voice from within you whispers, "At least see what the next step looks like!" are you able to listen to yourself and get out of your way?

That was exactly what I did: I listened to myself, and then I began taking the next exploratory steps. The process itself was validating and affirming; it served as a reminder that this life is mine to live and that I have the capacity to live it with as much intention and purpose as I possibly can.

The decision to move forward with the creation of WeGot-This.org was every bit as important as the decision to pick myself up and continue fighting my cancer, but something fundamental had shifted within me. Something had expanded.

In the moment I said yes to the idea of the nonprofit, I also said yes to shifting my mindset and redefining my relationship with cancer. No longer would I just be fighting my cancer; I'd be *living my life* with a renewed sense of purpose, connection, and control. I am fighting cancer, and I am also living with purpose. The two things are not mutually exclusive. I can do both at once.

On that same day, I called my CPA, told him what I was thinking about, and asked him to start thinking about what a project like this would look like in a finite, figures-on-paper sense. What would be required, and what steps would need to be taken to turn this from an abstract idea into a full-fledged reality?

From our spare bedroom that day, the idea of WeGotThis.org was born. On that same day, the darkness that had been weighing me down, robbing me of breath, began to lift. It not only lifted; it also transformed.

The darkness became light.

Collaboration Comes Alive

Obviously, teamwork and collaboration are vital forces in my life.

In a very real way, you and I are forming a new team, too. A fresh collaboration. As our journey progresses, my hope is that the stories I share and the insights I pass along will awaken something inside you—whether it's a goal, a dream, or a renewed sense of purpose and direction. I'm hopeful that you can weave even a small thread of my shared wisdom and experiences into the fabric of your daily life in a way that feels most comfortable, most authentic, and most applicable to you. That's what collaboration is all about: shared energy with the expectation of a positive outcome.

For me, collaboration also brings clarity. There were many moments when the very idea and concept of WeGotThis.org came into greater focus with stunning (and sometimes sudden) clarity. As the idea itself began to take shape and move toward becoming a reality, I relied on—and actively solicited—the counsel and guidance of those who could add fuel to this growing flame.

I want to share some of the singular moments that helped bring the organization into being. This, to me, is creative collaboration at its very, very best.

The Gasp

Alex and Alexa Karsos are dear friends of mine and old college buddies. Alex, who has experience in both tech and with start-ups (which I definitely don't), gamely and graciously offered to have weekly calls with me as I was sorting through the idea of starting this project.

As I was sharing my vision with them of how this entity would allow cancer patients to select the products they needed to make their lives more comfortable, Alex broke in with a question that brought everything into focus: "You mean it would be kind of like a baby registry?" he asked.

Alexa and I both gasped.

With that one simple, clarifying question, the picture of WeGotThis.org emerged on a blank canvas in full, vivid color. It almost felt like watching a black-and-white photo develop into full color. A little stunned by Alex's clarity, I still remember my response:

"Well, no, that's not exactly what I meant, Alex . . . but your description is even *better*!"

The parallel with the baby registry was spot-on! What was also inspiring was the fact that this clarity about a cancer-focused platform was coming from a noncancer person—proof positive that collaborative energy like this has no boundaries or limits.

That single moment, that single question—"You mean it would be kind of like a baby registry?"—was defining and definitely gasp-worthy. It helped set us on our way.

The Evolution

During a photo shoot some time ago, while we were creating a series of video interviews with our volunteers and supporters, a good friend made a simple statement that pulled everything about WeGoThis.org into a single, beautiful image. It felt like I'd been peering through a kaleidoscope and suddenly watched all the brightly colored fragments fall together into a single, beautiful shape. He reflected on how our organization was single-handedly creating an **evolution of giving**.

"I feel like we've created a *movement* that's totally redefining and expanding the act of giving and receiving, especially giving and receiving during difficult, challenging times. We're creating an evolution of giving, Elissa!" he said.

He was exactly right: People readily and happily give and receive gifts during joyous, celebratory events—a bridal shower, a baby shower, a birthday, a wedding. But what happens to our giving and sharing sensibilities during the *difficult* times? We don't even like *talking* about the things we want and need when we're going through a dark period; it almost feels like we're whining, complaining, or asking for a charitable handout.

I am immensely proud of the fact that WeGotThis.org has, indeed, created an *evolution of giving*. By creating a marketplace and a gift registry from which patients and their supporters can select the products and items that will bring them the most comfort and joy, we're affirming that we *do* have a choice. We *do* know how to communicate our needs effectively. And we *can* create an environment where giving and receiving can be done compassionately and purposefully, not just in the happy times but in the not-so-happy times as well. In fact, *especially* in the not-so-happy times.

The List

Yet another source of creative, collaborative energy—and this was even before I began thinking about starting the nonprofit—was Dr. Julia Bruckner, Ellie's pediatrician since the day she was born. She's still her pediatrician and a big part of her life. In fact, during Ellie's first year of life, we saw Dr. Bruckner more often than most of my own family and friends! Dr. Bruckner remains a close friend and a trusted voice of knowledge, insight, and wisdom.

When I was first diagnosed, Dr. Bruckner shared a bit of indispensable foresight: "People are going to be asking you how they can help, and I know you're going to say that you don't need anything, Elissa, but make a list of the things you think you'll need or want during treatment. You can even give your list to Eric so that when people ask what you need, he can respond, on your behalf, with specificity and intention."

She was right on all fronts, of course. When people learned of my diagnosis, they *did* ask me what I wanted, and I *did* usually say something innocuous, such as, "Oh, nothing in particular. Just your positive energy is enough." I also *didn't* want to make a list of items that would make my life a little easier because, to me, the gesture felt a little empty. It felt inappropriate and needy, simply because I'd been conditioned—as we all have, particularly women—to believe that clearly communicating about one's needs, particularly during challenging times, is unseemly. It felt like I was waiting for a handout.

I followed her advice. Creating the list was instructive and inspiring—not just for me, as it allowed me to clarify and communicate what I wanted and needed to make my life more comfortable as a cancer patient, but also for Eric, in his role as conduit and advocate, and for the gift givers themselves. It gave them the information and direction they needed to purchase products that I'd selected myself, products that I knew I could really *use*. A true win-win-win.

In short, the list itself filled an important gap in the gift-giving and give-receiving dynamic.

I never forgot Dr. Bruckner's guidance. In fact, it is the cornerstone of everything we represent: choice, freedom, and community.

The Momentum Begins . . . and Builds and Builds

Without the talent, resources, and creative energy from my earliest supporters, we would not be what (and where) we are today.

Along every single step of this journey, it has been one extraordinary human being after another, one amazing organization after another, and one fiercely dedicated volunteer working side by side with another that has kept our collective flame burning brightly.

The people who were placed in my path at the very outset of this journey—those first supporters—have helped influence its growth, its trajectory, and its tremendously positive impact.

All our supporters, volunteers, and advocates play a vital role; each person brings unique talent, resources, and genuine love for everything we are trying to achieve. But it was the early buy-in from our very first supporters that helped chart our overall course— those people and organizations that recognized at the outset the powerful, positive force for good that we would bring to the cancer community. (I'm convinced that the reason they "got it" so quickly is that they already know what "good" looks like.) They are powerful, positive forces in the world in their own right.

When I was first getting the organization off the ground, one of those "forces" was Geraldine "Gerri" Randlett, who was my class dean when I was a student at Babson College in Wellesley, Massachusetts. She's not just a force but also a *force of nature.*

Gerri, AVP of Alumni Engagement and Annual Giving at Babson College, is the person, the force of nature, the "electric current" who created the connection between me and the very first supporters of WeGotThis.org, all of whom hail from Babson themselves!

Gerri maintains close, intimate connections with Babson alumni all over the world; she seems to have a finger on every pulse and always knows what we're up to. Equally important, she's amazing at creating connections and potential partnerships among Babson alumni to create a greater good in the world. She was the glue—or, more accurately, a *magnet*—that brought me together with two Babson alumni who ended up adding invaluable support to this mission.

I'd already developed what I would describe as an "intimate affinity" for Bombas socks long before I was even thinking about the nonprofit. Early in my chemo, I suffered from occasional infections in the cuticles of my toenails, a fairly common occurrence. Keeping my feet warm during the chemo was also a challenge. I needed a well-made sock that could help with both issues.

The fact that Bombas socks don't have seams (which eliminates the constant friction of a seam rubbing against the toes) was a game changer. Because the socks are well made and super-comfortable, they also kept my feet warm and cozy during chemo in a way that less expensive socks simply could not.

Gerri put me in contact with two of the Bombas founders, Andrew Heath and David Heath, and we spent time talking through the concept and the goals of my nonprofit. Their support came very quickly thereafter. Their early involvement back then and their constant, unyielding support today make all the difference.

Today we are able to offer discount codes for Bombas on our website, and in return Bombas donates a percentage of those sales back to WeGotThis.org. Having access to items such as these brings *specific* comfort to cancer patients as they navigate the ups and downs of cancer treatment—a fact to which I can personally and passionately attest!

But their support didn't come automatically, simply by virtue of the fact that we were all Babson alums. Yes, the Babson connection definitely helped open the door to that initial exploratory conversation, but what informed their decision to move forward and create a collaborative synergy was the fact that they believed in the idea. They shared my belief that it would bring benefit and comfort to those living with cancer and that it would bring greater good to the community.

As a brand, the "greater good" is something Bombas is constantly striving for: For every pair of socks purchased, the company makes an equal donation of socks to people experiencing homelessness. They work very closely with a number of organizations—like we do—that create equally positive energy in the world. They are serious about making the world a better place.

Another early (and ongoing) partner in comfort and giving was Crocs, Inc., the American footwear company that has changed the landscape of comfortable shoe apparel and redefined the notion of corporate philanthropy.

Thanks to Gerri, who connected me with Daniel Marques of Crocs (who, again, happens to be a Babson alumni), an initial conversation quickly blossomed into a fruitful, rejuvenating collaboration.

Crocs is also closely aligned with values that bring benefit, connection, and *comfort* to the world. It's what also drives and defines WeGotThis.org. We strive to create comfort in the midst of discomfort. It also doesn't hurt that Crocs are supercomfortable—and they're just plain fun.

Again, I will speak from my own experience as a cancer thriver: There were many times, particularly during the early rounds of chemo, when I *couldn't* wear shoes. It was too uncomfortable. I'd also have to apply ice packs to my feet, which was unpleasant and, well, cold. Even the simple act of getting up out of the chair and walking to the bathroom at the infusion center seemed, at times, insurmountable . . . until I got my first pair of Crocs. Then everything changed.

Crocs describes itself as a company that is "rooted in comfort" and "always invites the world to come as you are."

Our sentiments exactly.

WeGotThis.org encourages and invites cancer thrivers and their supporters to root themselves in comfort by surrounding themselves with the things they need to make their journey more joyful. We, too, invite those who are accessing our registry to "come to us" exactly as they are.

This alignment of values not only solidifies but also *defines* the collaborative spirit we all share together.

Collaboration, Not Competition

In many ways the decision to launch WeGotThis.org emerged organically and as the result of a burning need to fill the gaps in my own life. However, I also realized that starting such an organization would bring real value to the cancer community.

For many reasons and on many levels then, the decision to launch was a big one. That's why I was thorough in my research and purposeful in the preliminary steps I took, even during the initial exploratory stage.

I spent quite a bit of time and effort, for example, to make sure that there wasn't another organization already in the world that provided a nonprofit gift registry for cancer patients. I certainly didn't want to reinvent the wheel or duplicate already-existing efforts.

If there had been an organization that was already on the ground running, already providing the same services and choices that I wanted to provide, I would not have proceeded. Instead, I would have probably joined forces with that organization, offering them my time, my talent, my experience, and my creative energy so that we would be moving in the same direction and sharing the same goal rather than competing with each other. (I realize that nonprofits don't "compete," obviously, but it is possible for nonprofits with similar goals and missions to end up taking resources from one another, whether intentionally or not. I wasn't interested in creating a competitive landscape. I didn't want that to happen. If there had been an existing platform with a nonprofit gift registry for cancer patients, I'd have shown up there, too.)

But there wasn't. The field was open, and the need was there.

From the very beginning, it was important for WeGotThis. org to be structured as a nonprofit rather than a for-profit entity. The platform that we offer is free. We are not selling anything. We are not hawking our wares or trying to convince people to purchase certain products. We do not have "customers" and "clients." We are all part of the same community, constantly searching for ways to make life easier, happier, and just a little more comfortable for ourselves and each other.

I do this work because I believe in its positive impact. To the best of my ability, I want to ensure that each and every cancer thriver has the right to pursue and live a full, meaningful life. A life with choice. A life with purpose. A life that is rich, resonant, and happy.

Managing my nonprofit brings a sense of normalcy and purpose to my life as I balance navigating cancer with living as freely and fully as I possibly can. Without a doubt, it's a lot of hard work, but it doesn't feel like work at all. This is too much fun to be work.

As the organization grows, and as more and more people step up to offer their time, talent, financial resources, and simply willingness to make a difference, it serves as a powerful reminder that together, we can bring practical benefits and even happiness to the world around us. It's a powerful reminder that yes, people *do* want to come together to help each other, not just in the good times but also in the not-so-good times.

Creating WeGotThis.org changed the trajectory of my life not just by pulling me from the precipice of my own darkness but also by lifting me up, propelling me past my own pain, and steering me toward a higher ground and a greater good. Yes, I am still attentive to my cancer—I will be in treatment for the rest of my life—but I am also attentive to the larger world around me and to the precious moments that exist within each day, each hour, and every minute.

The "We" in "WeGotThis.org" is the world—and the concept—that drives everything.

I am not by myself. None of us are. When we come together, we become something else. When we come together, "I" becomes "We."

If that isn't a perfect enough reason to have started this organization, I don't know what is.

CHAPTER FIVE

REDEFINING SUCCESS

Make Your Own Metric

I want to share something I've uncovered about *success*: Pursuing and attaining it (success, that is) does not need to be a harrowing, stress-filled, anxiety-ridden, all-or-nothing experience.

Quite the opposite.

The pursuit of success, in my mind, is a constant journey of exploration, growth, discovery, and rediscovery. Just as we discussed in the opening chapters, as we run this race toward success, we have the freedom to change the location of our "finish line" at any given point.

If the nature and the course of our race shift, we have the power and the prerogative to either adjust course, take a breather, or, hell, create a bold, brave new course that involves dashing off into the woods where nobody expected us to go and where we never really expected to go ourselves. We are the final arbiters.

Each of us can have our own personal relationship with success. My definition of success isn't the same as yours, nor is yours the same as mine—or your partner's, your mother's, or your best friend's. Yes, there are common goals that most of us share, but even those must be interpreted and pursued in a way that feels the most comfortable and the most authentic to each of us in our own lives.

When it comes to success, *make your own metric, assume ownership,* and *exercise your option (and your right) as a human being to create the quality of life that you want and deserve.*

Contrary to popular opinion, there isn't some unyielding, preexisting yardstick lurking in your future, waiting to smack you in the head the moment you come up short. That's not the way it works. Not in my life, anyway.

Living with cancer—and facing the prospect of dying from it—has forced me to redefine the concept of success. Even though having cancer sucks, I am grateful that its arrival has pushed me toward a greater clarity about how the hell I want to make my way through my own life.

Your life is yours to live, and the *quality* of your life is yours to pursue, to nurture, and, ultimately, to control however you see fit.

A Wider View

If getting rid of cancer was my *only* benchmark for success, then I am fairly certain I would not be writing this book today. I wouldn't have the strength. Or the will. Or the desire. I would probably be too subsumed by the disease itself or, perhaps more accurately, too debilitated by the course of treatment we'd selected at that time, to be able to pick up a pen or move my fingers across a keyboard.

I want to be clear: I am deeply grateful that we decided on the treatment that we did, *when* we did because it was the right course of action at the time. The treatment itself—a cocktail of chemo-therapy combined with immunotherapy—was successful at shrinking many of my tumors and keeping the cancer at bay. I am alive today because of it.

But after several months in, I realized I couldn't allow myself to continue to accept that singular definition of success. The mind-blowingly powerful rounds of chemo were wearing me down and wiping me out.

Yes, the treatment was doing its job, and in a *clinical* sense, it was indeed successful because it was preventing the spread of the disease. However, what had become untenable and tortuous was the quality of life that I had been reduced to.

I was nauseous more often than not. Many days I couldn't get out of bed or even lift my head. I didn't have the energy to mean-ingfully engage with my two-year-old daughter, Ellie, or have a peaceful, pleasant, vomit-free dinner (yes, I said it) with my husband, Eric.

Every ounce of my physical and mental focus was concen-trated on staying alive and tolerating the meds—meds not only toxic enough to wipe out many of my tumors but also toxic enough to eradicate my happiness, my joy, and unravel every single thread of contentment and comfort I had. It was too much.

Even though I was succeeding at one thing—staying alive—I was failing miserably at another—enjoying my life while staying alive. I was failing in my effort to ensure a quality of life that was engaging, meaningful, and balanced. I'd reached a point where I was no longer willing to sacrifice one thing (staying alive) for another (being happy and fulfilled while I'm alive).

In a very real way, my success in one area of life was contributing to my failure in another, and I simply wasn't willing to continue living with the imbalance. That was when I made the decision to change treatments—a risky decision but one that ultimately paid off.

Because now I have my life back. My full life back. As a result of that very risky but very rewarding decision to find another course and change directions with my treatment, I was able to reconfigure my own definition of success.

I pick my daughter up from preschool, and I go to concerts with my husband. I run a thriving nonprofit that helps other cancer thrivers. I spend meaningful time with my family and friends, and I wake up each morning ready—and able—to get at it. I have created balance where there was once an intolerable imbalance. *I am succeeding.*

Today I define success by the quality and caliber of my own life, as well as the quality, caliber, and character of the people with whom I choose to interact. Healthy relationships are vital; I don't have the time or energy to be involved in toxic or unhealthy partnerships of any kind. If I am struggling with a toxic relationship, wasting precious time trying to right a wrong that will never be righted, or aligning myself with someone's values that simply don't align with mine, then I am falling short of my definition of success.

This unencumbered thinking comes from having developed a more expansive view, not just of my own life but also of the world around me. If I were to lay a single metric over all the nuanced layers of my life, I'd be doing myself a grave disservice.

I am worthy of more than a single metric.

When I think about how both my view and my vision have become wider since my diagnosis, I can't help but think of a quote from Van Gogh that has stuck with me ever since high school: "The important thing is to breathe as hard as ever we can breathe."

The Greatest Setbacks Can Yield the Greatest Success

Experiencing a major setback is a real drag. Coming face-to-face with failure is no fun. It reminds me of how my financial advising clients would feel during a market downturn. Losing hurts more than the joy of winning. In fact, there is a psychological term in finance built around this idea of "loss aversion." People experience losses more intensely than gains of the same size.

The good news is that your setbacks don't have to set you *all* the way back; they don't have to send you limping back to the starting gate with your tail between your legs. On the contrary. If you've cultivated a healthy outlook and a positive mindset, then what could be waiting for you on the other side of that setback is *success*, in the form of growth, resilience, and empowerment.

Our detours and "failures"—as humiliating and discouraging as they may feel in the moment—can eventually lead us in a new direction, down an untraveled path, toward opportunities and adventures we never could have imagined even existed. Sometimes *getting* to that new path can be painful, though—figuratively and literally. I speak from experience.

I'm going to return to my love of field hockey to help me make my point here. In the opening chapters, I reflected on how the sport nurtured within me that spirit of resilience, unrelenting drive, and a heightened sense of collective accountability—teamwork and togetherness at their absolute best. I played competitively in high school and college, and I loved everything about the sport.

However, two major roadblocks arose in the form of two major injuries: In the spring of my freshman year of college, I sustained a torn meniscus and ACL, which sidelined me for months. The following year I tore my shoulder labrum.

Those injuries represented the biggest setbacks I'd ever experienced in my life. Before that, I'd never encountered anything quite as devastating. It felt like my world was crashing down around me . . . or at least crumbling at an accelerated rate. In those moments I simply couldn't see the silver linings that were waiting for me, even though many were to come.

In the days and weeks following the injuries and surgeries, I remember asking myself questions that didn't yet have answers: How long will it take my body to bounce back so that I can get back out there on the field? Will I still be in top form once I'm back? What happens if I'm not as good as I used to be?

As the answers began to reveal themselves, I was faced with an awful moment of truth: I *was* struggling out there on the field, and I *was* falling short of the athletic excellence that I—and equally important, my teammates—had come to expect and rely on.

It was my parents, though, who posed the single question that helped change the course of my trajectory, not only in field hockey but also in my larger life. The way they asked it didn't make me feel small, defeated, broken, or even bent, for that matter. If anything, their question opened a new door in my mind—a door that had not only been closed to me before but one I never even knew existed. They looked at me, could see that I was struggling, and simply asked,

"Do you **have** to keep playing, Elissa?"
As soon as they asked me, the answer bubbled up from within me immediately. "No, I don't really have to continue playing at all."

It wasn't a question of whether I'd miss it. Yes, I'd miss everything about field hockey—the camaraderie, the competition, the collective focus, and the physical rigors of the game itself. It was a question of whether I could stop playing—and walk away. I knew that my injuries had compromised my performance to the extent that my staying on the team would have diminished the overall competitive abilities of the team, which was untenable. They wouldn't have enjoyed it. I wouldn't have enjoyed it. Walking away was the best choice.

But here's the thing about "walking away": The moment you begin walking away from one thing, you begin walking toward something fresh and unknown—even if it doesn't feel like it at the time.

Perhaps my choice of words isn't quite as accurate as it could be: I didn't really "walk toward" an exciting new experience; I *flew* toward it—literally.

In my junior year of college, after deciding to stop playing field hockey for good, I also decided to explore my interest in marketing and PR. So I boarded a plane to Los Angeles to begin an internship with a music performing rights organization called BMI. That was when my life opened up in just about every conceivable way.

I was suddenly living in a new place—on UCLA's campus, no less!—far away from home, school, family, and friends. For the first time in my adult life, I was developing meaningful professional relationships with people in a work setting. The people at BMI supported me, they gladly shared their wisdom, and they wanted to see me succeed. I completely immersed myself in the experience.

That was when things clicked for me, and I began to recognize the power of networking and the joy of creating circles of people around me who were willing to teach me, show me the ropes, and, perhaps unwittingly, become an important part of my successful career trajectory. Had I remained on the field hockey team, or had I not believed in myself enough to chart a new course, I wouldn't be where I am today, living the full life that I live. My parents' question gave me the freedom to look at new possibilities beyond what I had "always done" when the circumstances changed.

The lesson here is that walking away from one thing doesn't *always* dictate that you'll walk toward something new. You've got to *create* the opportunity. You've got to pick yourself up after you've stumbled (or, in my case, torn your shoulder and ACL). You've got to steer your life onto a new path, even if you're unsure where it will lead. Sometimes "enough is enough" when you are pounding sand and feeling sorry for yourself.

Learning to listen to the people around you whom you love and trust, even if they're telling you something you might not necessarily want to hear, is sometimes necessary. Your ability to hear them doesn't mean you must always follow their direction. In fact, remember when a handful of well-meaning loved ones urged me not to start the nonprofit while undergoing chemo? Well, I didn't listen. The decisions you make about how you want to pursue your own success and navigate your own life belong to you and you alone.

Even though I knew deep down in my heart that my time as a field hockey player had come to an end, I'm grateful that I had the capacity to really listen to the question my parents posed to me during that difficult time: "Do you **have** to keep playing, Elissa?" Because the answer that came back to me—"No, I don't!"—is what set me on my new path.

These are the places where true success really lives.

Fly, Elissa, Fly

By the time I returned to school for my senior year after the LA internship, I was not at all stressed out by the fact that I didn't have a job lined up when I graduated. I had something better: Confidence. Drive. A new vision of myself and my capabilities. Equally important, I had friends now who lived in LA and who were in the music industry. I had contacts!

My definition of success had expanded exponentially. No longer would it be measured by the number of wins on the field but by how effectively I could maximize my experience in LA and transform it into something more than just a summer internship. I felt like I had wings, and I used them to fly back to LA. After graduating, I bought a one-way plane ticket and flew toward my continually unfolding career in the entertainment industry. I called everyone I knew from my days as an intern and secured my first full-time job in fairly short order as an executive assistant to the CEO of the then music publishing company Bug Music. My former boss at my internship at BMI helped steer me to my first full-time, paid position. I was on my way.

After learning a tremendous amount about the industry and meeting extraordinarily talented people, many of whom remain close friends, my career interests expanded and took yet another turn. I made a fresh leap into the world of corporate sales—a move that would heighten my ascension, invigorate my earning potential, and bolster my self-confidence. I was evolving into the person I was to become.

Sales was exciting and rewarding on many different levels. Within the first fiscal year, I was making a healthy six-figure salary, winning every promotional prize I could win, and breaking every record that could be broken—a long way from my days as an injured field hockey player or even my early days in LA as an executive assistant barely making $30,000 a year. Most important? I was happy. Fulfilled. Stimulated. Comfortable. *Complete.*

I share this sequence of events from my early adult life to make the point that I didn't just accidentally stumble onto a successful career path. I *made* it happen, along with the counsel, support, and guidance of the people I knew and trusted in my rapidly expanding circle. *We* made it happen together.

In my world, as you already know, it's all about the "we."

This brief glimpse into my early adulthood is proof positive that success—not just finding it but searching for it, too—cannot happen in an isolated vacuum. Both the pursuit and the attainment of success require input and gentle steering from the people around you, too, whether those people are family members, friends, employers, potential employers, or maybe even just the one random stranger who ends up becoming a friend after a brief, positive encounter.

All these key people in your life—the ones you know well and the ones you're just getting to know—can have a powerful, positive impact on how your life unfolds, on the success you achieve, and on the life you live. All these things help enrich, deepen, and define the quality of your life, which, for me, is everything.

Although I don't want to undermine the importance of making money and living well, I do want to emphasize that part of "living well" is composed of a comfortable, connective quality of life. Without that, all else is empty.

The people who surround you can help create a positive orbit as you step into new spaces and embark on new journeys. I speak from experience. The people in my "orbit"—whether it's my team of doctors, my family and friends, the volunteers who give so much to WeGotThis.org, or the woman sitting beside me in the infusion room as we both receive our treatments—are all instrumental in creating various levels of success in my life. They are more than instrumental, in fact. All these healthy relationships *make my life successful.*

I am living on my own terms, and that is my definition of success. I do not need to be in remission to experience this thing called success. I do not need to be cured to be happy and complete. My life today is full, and equally important, it is *fun*. This is what I call a "win." This is what I call success.

As you make your own metrics for success, be honest with yourself. Be gentle, wise, and loving with yourself, too. Try your best to surround yourself with people who share the same passions, the same values, and the same sense of purpose and integrity as you do.

I'm happy to say that I am not just striving toward success, yearning for it, or hoping for it.

I am also *living* it.

Every single day of my life.

CHAPTER SIX

DIFFICULT MOMENTS

Moving Through Moments of Darkness

I try to be very deliberate and intentional when I'm talking (or writing) about cancer, particularly my own cancer, because I never want to romanticize my diagnosis.

I do have cancer . . . but I also happen to have what many would describe as, well, a cheerful disposition and an energetic, "can do" sensibility.

I've *always* been optimistic and forward moving; it's built into my DNA. I am not swimming (or drowning) in the waters of denial, but I'm also not basking in the sun for any longer than is appropriate. What I *am* doing, though, is standing smack dab in the center of my life, cherishing each and every moment. Even the moments that are uncomfortable and painful.

Yes, the fact that I have terminal cancer really blows, but the bottom line is that my diagnosis is distinct from my disposition. I am not cancer. I only *have* cancer.

When I'm facing a roadblock or a detour, or when I receive a call from my oncologist (like I did recently) telling me that my cancer has returned in certain areas, I try to remind myself that the moment itself will soon be over. Whenever I'm in the middle of a dark, difficult situation that can sometimes obscure the sight of the sun, I try to remind myself that once I get through it and to the other side, I will still be me.

This way of thinking and living doesn't mean that I'm blinded by my own optimism. Far from it. My diagnosis has only magnified the clarity with which I see myself and the world around me. In fact, having cancer opened my mind and heart even wider to the idea that even in the darkest moments, there is light. When there isn't light, I know there will be because that light will come from me. I will create it.

Nothing is more illuminating than the kind of light that shines from the inside of a silver lining.

From the moment I found out I had cancer, I desperately needed to find a silver lining in this experience. The journey itself is challenging enough. I needed to create the opportunity to redefine it from my own perspective.

It was important to me, especially in those early stages, to find something bright that would come out of the darkness. To create that silver lining to make my life with cancer more manageable, more bearable, and more empowering. Happier.

I felt the need to find purpose out of my cancer experience, so I didn't dwell in the negativity of why I got it in the first place. I had to create something that was bigger than me and my single experience. I wanted to fill the gaps that I fell into during my diagnosis. When I came up with the initial idea for my nonprofit, it breathed a whole new life into me. I felt a legacy forming that I was proud of. I found the light in the darkness not because it suddenly appeared but because I *created* it. Today WeGotThis.org shines bright into the lives of cancer thrivers all over the country who are in need of resources and choices that will help make their lives a little easier and more comfortable.

As we explored in the previous chapter, my nonprofit keeps me driven and highly focused. It propels me. I *want* to work hard every single day to make this gift registry for cancer patients as vibrant and diverse as possible. In a very real way, the work that I do to create choices for cancer patients helps *this* cancer patient—me!—feel more alive and connected.

In our busy daily lives, this kind of conscious contemplation is not often considered a priority. But when times get tough and days get dark, we really need to have a source of comfort and relief. It's best not to wait until you need it. Create it *before* you need it.

I also want to be careful about oversimplifying the concept of silver linings. I don't want to leave the impression that there is only one per customer or only one per crisis. Being able to navigate difficult moments with grace and dignity requires a more holistic approach.

When I was first diagnosed, I started playing golf almost every day, which was not only great exercise and a healthy, much-needed distraction but also *fun*. It made—and still makes—me happy. It brings balance to my life. Before cancer, I was an avid tennis player, but it became too high impact during my initial chemo rounds. Picking up golf gave me an accessible sport to play, no matter how sick I was, and that familiarity gave me a lot of comfort. Having activities and experiences (even if they were slightly different from what I was used to) that could bring me joy during the darkest days helped me prioritize the value of living life.

My chemo infusions were typically three weeks apart. For about two weeks after each infusion, I experienced all the stereotypical symptoms: throwing up, loss of taste, mouth sores, and yes, I was bald. But for a few days before the start of the next round, I would feel like myself again. I would get this window of time where I felt empowered and grateful to be me.

I'm lucky that the people in my life also helped me feel like myself again. Eric's presence in my life is *everything*. Particularly when I was first beginning treatment, having Eric by my side—taking me to doctor's appointments, helping me navigate the complexities of the sometimes indecipherable medical jargon, fluffing my pillow when I could barely lift my head, and showering our daughter, Ellie, with pure, parental love that felt like it was coming from both of us (the list could fill the pages of this book)—brought me happy, healing energy when I needed it most. Even when I didn't feel like my best self (or even me at all), Eric showed up to remind me I was. Who I was—the core of myself— was unchanged.

He would know the timeline of my symptoms better than I did. I would be frustrated by how much my mouth hurt from my tongue feeling like sandpaper, and he would remind me that I was on day three of my chemo cycle, and it should subside within a few days. I would start to feel down and like everything was caving in, but he would remind me that this would always happen at my most painful parts of the recovery. It was his *constant* presence by my side during those early months that helped save my life. It is his continued support and alignment that help keep me alive and living a full, balanced life to this very day.

Difficult Decisions

When you're diagnosed with cancer, you're forced to make a lot of very difficult decisions very quickly: which treatments you'll pursue, which doctors you'll see, which hospital you'll commute to. Imagine only having a twelve-hour window to decide if you'll ever want to have more children.

Immediately following the doctor giving me the malignant biopsy results, the hospital prioritized talking with a fertility specialist. It wasn't a matter of insurance (everything would be covered), and it wasn't a matter of doctor availability (mine rushed to see me that same day). It was a matter of timing. It was not at an ideal time in my cycle when I found out that I had cancer. I hadn't even processed the fact that I had breast cancer yet, but I had to decide by that evening at nine o'clock if I was going to start the hormone shots to freeze my eggs. Even if I started, there were no guarantees, but it was the choice of whether or not I wanted to go into chemo knowing that I had tried everything possible to preserve my future fertility. I appreciated that they put a focus on this and valued it for our family, but that's not a choice that's ever easy to make, let alone make in the hours after a massive cancer diagnosis!

Many people have cancer, do chemo, and continue having children. This wasn't the case for me because I'm stage IV. I cannot safely take a long enough break from chemo to either go through IVF or get pregnant naturally and wait out a full-term pregnancy. I would die. The cancer would kill me.

Having a stage IV cancer diagnosis within a year of having your first child is horrifying for a number of reasons, but the idea of having to go through fertility treatments again, so soon, was the last straw for me. After having endometriosis since the eighth grade, getting pregnant was challenging enough already. We had opted for an intrauterine insemination, which worked the first time but was not a viable pregnancy. It took some time for my body to get back to a place where we could try again. But we did and had a successful pregnancy with our daughter, Ellie.

I didn't cry when I found out my biopsies were malignant. I didn't cry when I found out there was more cancer in my liver than in my breast. I didn't even cry at my wedding. However, being forced to decide whether I would ever have children again while also making sure that I will be around for my current child, well, that's just fucked up. I broke down.

After nearly three years of trying to get pregnant and after a miscarriage, we had the most perfect baby in the middle of the pandemic. In July 2020 our daughter, Ellie, was born, and the world shut down. We always pictured having another child, but who knows what we would have ultimately decided. We thought we had time to make that choice: contemplating a sibling, spending a few years deciding, picking out gender neutral colors in case our next one was a boy. All that was deemed unnecessary within a single day.

There are plenty of other ways to grow a family, and I think they're all wonderful options. But this wasn't just about conceiving ourselves; it was also about whether to grow our family while the odds are that I won't live a full life. This was heavy shit.

I brought home all the hormone shots, buying myself as much time in case I chose to start the egg freezing process. I looked at Eric and asked, "Can you be okay with me not wanting to do this?" We had an hour left to decide. I knew that taking away the possibility of another child was heartbreaking. I worried he would beg me to do it, to keep our options open.

"Of course," he replied. "All I want is for you to be okay."

We won't have more children because that's the choice we've made with the hand we've been dealt. I will pour all my time and energy into Ellie and her growth and happiness. I have a limited amount of energy each day, as do we all, and I made a decision to commit it all to her. Maybe I would have made that decision without cancer. We'll never know. But I know where we are now, and I believe it's the right place for us.

Am I mad that cancer took so much from me? Yes. I fucking hate cancer. Cancer sucks. But rather than dwelling on the fact that I can't have more biological children without risking my life, I choose to focus on how incredibly lucky I am that we already had Ellie. I get to be with her for the rest of my life.

Making that choice was extraordinarily challenging, and I'm extraordinarily lucky I had the right people in my life to help give me guidance. Because my doctor was so helpful in informing and counseling me, I thought I'd cede some space here that she might do the same for anyone struggling with the same hard choice and asked my amazing fertility specialist Dr. Alison Peck, Board Certified Reproductive Endocrinologist, to share her insights directly:

Hope for the Future

There are not many opportunities in life where a stranger in need calls and you drop everything to help because you know that's the right thing to do. As a fertility doctor, that's what I do when I get the cancer diagnosis phone call from a patient. And that's what I did with Elissa.

Among my many roles as a reproductive endocrinologist and fertility specialist, the one I hold most dear is giving women the opportunity to preserve their eggs for future use. Eggs are precious gems. And before chemotherapy or reproductive surgery, it is important to pause and ask yourself, what can I do to give myself hope to have a future family or extended family?

Today it has been commonplace for women to freeze eggs to "stop the biological clock." But the original intention of egg freezing was to preserve eggs for cancer patients. Cancer treatment can diminish or prevent a women's ability to have biological children by killing eggs or diminishing ovarian hormone production and function. By freezing a group of eggs before starting treatment, patients can return after successful treatment and resume their family building.

When I get the call in the brief window of time between someone's cancer diagnosis and treatment, a fast-forward button is pushed to start fertility medications right away and harvest some eggs. It takes approximately two weeks. Many companies in the fertility industry have rallied to help with medications and to curb the cost of treatment.

From my physician perspective, the most important place I can help in the cancer patient's journey is to give hope for a bright future. Giving someone the opportunity to save eggs is really giving them a reason to fight and to maintain their ability to create a future life. That's what egg freezing in cancer patients means to me. Whether or not someone chooses to freeze their eggs, giving them a moment to make that choice is crucial. I want every cancer patient to know this and have their moment to decide.

Glorious Growth

When we move through moments of darkness—and by "we" I don't just mean Eric and me but all of us collectively, including you—our resilience grows. Our adaptability awakens. We become more warrior like. Our "badass" quotient rises exponentially. We might not feel all this growth and maturation as it is happening, but trust me, it is happening.

By-products can emerge from adversity and challenge. Difficult moments don't have to just be difficult moments.

If nothing positive results from this cancer I happen to have, it would mean that **all I have is cancer**, and that doesn't work for me. My life is more than cancer. It must be. And it is.

I want to return to this concept of growth during adversity and how awesome it is to tap into—and witness—our own adaptability and resilience while navigating a difficult life detour or an uncomfortably bumpy path.

When we were first presented with the results of my PET scan as we sat together in the surgeon's office, Eric and I stared at the screen showing my body covered in lights. Those little pinpricks lit up like a morbid Christmas tree.

The moment itself was shocking, of course, but Eric and I reacted quite differently to what we had just seen. I immediately went into my practical, problem-solving, what-do-we-have-to-do-to-beat-this-thing mode, but Eric's shock rendered him silent and still. It was the first time we'd actually seen a physical image of the disease that was raging throughout my body, the first time we were able to visually track its aggressive movement. It was the first time we were told that my cancer was stage IV.

Since that blinding "lights everywhere" moment, though, Eric's shock has both dissolved *and* evolved. It has transformed and grown into something else.

Certainly, that raw moment of realization *needed* to happen, and I'm glad it did. However, the passage of time and accumulation of knowledge (Eric knows virtually everything there is to know about stage IV metastatic breast cancer—far more than I do, that's for sure) has brought with it a far greater sense of control and confidence and, with it, resilience.

Today, though, my cancer isn't blinding. It's far from the only thing we see. We are certainly attentive to it and mindful of its presence, but our lives are also filled with other things—projects, people, and passions that are near and dear to our hearts. Even though my cancer is showing signs of returning, and we will take whatever steps necessary to keep kicking its ass, we will continue to remain closely aligned with the principles that define us. Even if darkness descends—and it will, occasionally, because that's just part of life—we will stick close to the stuff we love.

Become a Safe Haven

I am extremely fortunate to have a *multitude* of safe havens available to me and equally fortunate to function as a safe haven to a multitude of people who also need a peaceful harbor themselves. I want to share and celebrate a few of my safe havens here, beginning with this story:

It was just a few days before Ellie's first birthday when I received the phone call telling me I have cancer. From there, everything happened very fast: The debilitating chemo. The endless doctor's visits (and fighting like hell to make sure those visits happened as timely as possible, which was a challenge in itself). The upsetting lack of energy. The all-consuming nausea. The waves of stress and anxiety that washed over me and Eric as we tried to care for our daughter in a way that shielded her from our fear of the unknown.

Two very dear friends became our safe haven during those first few months: a lovely, loving couple who became members of my boxing gym almost as soon as it opened and were deeply involved with and strongly supportive of (and generous to) our nonprofit.

They would often swing by to watch Ellie when I was too sick to get out of bed. They'd come to check on me, of course, but they'd also come to help with whatever I needed help with (particularly when Eric was out at a gig) and to simply hang out with Ellie while I rested.

One afternoon, when Eric was on the road and I was so sick I could barely move, they came over with their two daughters in tow and demanded that I hightail it to my bedroom to rest. They'd also arrived bearing precious gifts, not only lunch but also a beautiful dollhouse for Ellie!

I'll never forget how comforted I was by their presence that day. Even as I rested—even in my *sleep*—I felt tremendous relief, just knowing they were hanging out with Ellie, showering her with love, and introducing her to her new dollhouse. I remember how the sound of their laughter (Ellie's included!) made me smile in my sleep.

Although countless other friends and family members offered similar support (and still offer it today), the memory of that beautiful "dollhouse visit" has always remained with me.

What I appreciated most was not just the presents they brought but also their *presence* that day. They weren't intrusive; their presence didn't feel forced or weighty. (Sidenote: Learning to be present for someone you love without being overbearing is definitely an art, and in my opinion it's one of the most important skills a human being can have, particularly in a time of crisis or need.)

This is one of the many reasons I loved them like I did: They knew, instinctively, when I needed them, but they also had the wisdom and the discernment to reach out and call me or Eric beforehand to ask "Listen, could you use a visit? If not, we'll stay home, but if so, we're on our way!"

This beautiful family had mastered the art of "being there" to the point of perfection or as close to perfection as one could get—a vital skill during dark times.

But cancer crawled into their lives, too.

Right around the time COVID-19 slammed into the world, the mom was diagnosed with breast cancer. She has beaten it back and lives today as a survivor and a warrior.

About a year after my own diagnosis, the husband was also diagnosed with cancer. He fought it like hell. He fought it like the trooper and the warrior he was. After a time, though, the cancer became too aggressive and uncontrollable. I received a phone call one sunny afternoon letting me know that he was in the hospital and that things were not looking so great.

I hightailed it to the hospital, of course, but not without calling first to see if my presence would be welcome—a lesson I had learned from them. I remember sitting with the family in the ICU, waiting room as doctors and family members filed in and out. I know, beyond the shadow of a doubt, that my presence that day made a difference to them. I know it in my heart. Theirs had made a difference to me.

It made a difference to him, too. Lying in his hospital bed, hooked up to tubes and wires and barely able to keep his eyes open, I remember leaning in close to tell him that I loved him and that he needed to get his butt back to the gym so that we could box together again. I am certain he heard me because even in the tangle of tubes and medical equipment surrounding him, I saw the shadow of a smile pass across his face.

He died a few days later.

In the days leading up to his funeral—as well as in those dark, difficult days right after the funeral, when the swirl of activity had settled down and the grief had been given room to settle in—I called and asked the family, "Hey, could you guys use some Ellie time?"

The answer was yes. They wanted to see my daughter, Ellie, and to feel the power and purity of her youthful energy and bright presence.

So Ellie and I went over for a visit. We sat together. We played. We spoke quietly. We even laughed a little. By then Ellie was about three and a half years old, so she'd become very vocal and engaging. That afternoon together, sitting in their living room, we were each other's safe havens.

I remember watching as the two sisters played with Ellie on their couch that afternoon. Then they made a pillow fort on the floor. As I watched them play, I thought back to that afternoon when we were all together at *my* home, during my time of need, how they'd brought over the dollhouse and created those moments of joy and comfort for each other and for me as well, as I rested in bed, listening to their happy sounds.

Witnessing that simple scene, with Ellie sitting in between the two girls, provided stunning affirmation that safe havens are real. They're not just some feel-good, pie-in-the-sky concept designed to sprinkle fairy dust over everything. They don't have to be a place or a physical space. The stability and comfort of a safe haven are powerful and palpable. All of us have the power to create and nurture those safe havens so that they are there when we need them. Many times, the spoken word is not necessary at all. In times of grief or pain, the power and promise of a person's presence and proximity are enough. Sometimes they're everything.

When you're searching for ways to comfort someone who is grieving or navigating a difficult moment, saying the right thing in the right way isn't always necessary. Your mere presence can often be the greatest source of comfort during crisis. We can be each other's safe havens, even in silence. All of us can be. You can be, too.

The fact that I was there for this family when they needed me and that they were there for me in my time of need fills me with gratitude. I miss him tremendously, but I'm thankful to have been a part of his life. I'm thankful he was part of mine—along with Eric's and Ellie's. I see the results of his goodness and generosity each and every day. I see it in the positive impact his generosity has had on my nonprofit. I see it when I look at the beautiful humans his daughters are growing up to be. These are the things that endure.

When the waters get rough and the waves get high, it sure feels good to have a safe harbor and to know that there are people in your life who serve as a lighthouse in the storm, spreading light and standing as a beacon in the darkness. This is the kind of light that never really dims. I see and feel it whenever I watch Ellie play with her dollhouse.

Damn, I Look Good!

There's something unexpectedly awesome about feeling beautiful when you're in a tough spot or stuck in the middle of a crisis.

Perhaps it's the power that comes with being able to assume even a small degree of control at a time when all else around you seems to have slipped well beyond your grasp.

Getting dolled up and decked out, especially when you're having a bad day or facing a dark moment, is also just plain fun. It feels good. Simple as that.

A few weeks before I began chemo, a friend suggested I get my eyebrows microbladed; she had hers done just before her first round of chemo and loved the way it made her look and feel. (The process of microblading is just like it sounds: a technician uses tiny needles to tattoo eyebrows onto your face.)

I decided to go for it!

Since I was so close to the start date for my treatment, though, I had to get written clearance from my oncologist because the procedure of microblading brought with it the risk of infection. Luckily, my doctor confirmed that it was safe, so she sent a note, and I rushed in for my appointment.

Because time was of the essence—we needed to get this done quickly before my chemo began—the technician even agreed to have us meet her at her salon on a Sunday after she was normally closed. She was kind and generous enough to understand that this was a special request, without a moment to waste.

At first I was a little apprehensive and anxious about the microblading process, but I was apprehensive and anxious about my upcoming chemo, too, so I just figured, *What the hell?* Let me start with the process that will end up making me feel (and look) good!

On the Sunday evening before my chemo started, I went to the salon, and my friend made sure she was there to support me also. The technician first shaped my eyebrows so they were per-fect, and her friend microbladed them. We talked about the other things I was doing to prep for treatment, not the medical stuff but the fun stuff, such as wig shopping and cancer pun shirts. We confronted head-on the parts of myself that cancer might take away. I remember looking at myself in the mirror when I walked out of the salon, with my fancy new eyebrows, and thinking, *Damn, I look good!*

That evening of self-care and pampering not only brought me happiness in the moment, but it also helped get my mind right for the challenge that lay ahead. It bolstered my self-confidence and made me feel like I was ready for the chemo that was to come.

I still get lots of compliments on my eyebrows, even today. (I continue to maintain the microblading.)

On my cancer journey, I've had hair, and I haven't had hair. I've experienced both states of being. But the cancer never fully took away my eyebrows. Those are now permanently mine.

I'm not advocating microblading for everyone, of course. For me, it was empowering—a way to control the things I could con-trol in a way that brought me happiness and freedom. My hope is that you will prioritize the things that make you feel empowered, happy, and free.

Even More Choices

The sense of control I felt from that decision to microblade my eyebrows was really impactful for me. After that, I had other similar cosmetic choices to make, this time surrounding the hair on my head. When going into cancer treatment, I had the option to explore something called "cold capping," but I didn't know a lot about what it was. I basically knew it wouldn't be covered by insurance; it was very expensive and very, well, cold.

Cold capping is a way to lower the temperature of the head, which, in some cases, can reduce hair loss caused by chemo. Basically, the cold restricts blood flow, meaning that the amount of chemo that gets to the area (since it travels through the bloodstream) is reduced. Less chemo drugs can mean less damage to hair follicles—and less hair loss!

I knew other people who had tried it before, and while it wasn't guaranteed, it was a shot at keeping my hair. While I was curious about it, since hair loss is one of the most stereotypical symptoms of chemo, I ultimately decided not to do it. With stage IV cancer, it wouldn't be a permanent treatment solution. When I lost my hair with my initial cancer treatment, it was temporary and grew back. But I ended up losing my hair all over again with subsequent cancer therapies. So for me, cold capping wasn't the right move.

What was right for me was taking my hair loss into my own hands by proactively shaving it as it was falling out and embracing my new look. I wasn't someone who was comfortable with wigs or artificial hair. Instead, I wore a lot of beanies and rocked them in the way that felt most authentic to myself. And I felt incredibly empowered.

I've now been able to witness other people's experience and realize how personal a choice this is. My friend Jess, a vocalist who frequently tours with well-known artists, gave me a whole different perspective on just how personal and different it can be. Jess called me after seeing some of my Instagram posts and shared that she decided to check herself, finding a lump in her breast that was later diagnosed as breast cancer.

Jess currently performs with an artist who is known for huge tours. When Jess started looking into her treatment options, she had so many other things to consider. While I was worrying about whether my one-year-old might be scared of my bald head, Jess was worrying whether audiences of tens of thousands would recognize her bald head meant cancer. Being in the public eye, if she lost her hair to cancer treatment, the option whether to share her diagnosis would be automatically taken away. It wasn't something she wanted the world to know about yet. So for Jess, a treatment option such as cold capping made perfect sense. Many months after her treatment, she shared with me that while she still did lose most of her hair despite the cold capping, she was able to keep enough that she looked normal. Her decision helped her be her most authentic self throughout her cancer experience. After cancer treatment, Jess went on a huge tour and now continues to live her best life, not just physically but also emotionally.

I think it's pretty incredible that we can feel so empowered and authentically ourselves in totally opposite decisions during the same kind of hard time. Both choices are valid, and both were the right choice given who we are as individuals. Knowing ourselves and what will make us feel best in the hardest times isn't just important; it's also freeing.

Most people probably think that living with a terminal disease is anything but freeing, that living with stage IV metastatic breast cancer would be limiting and confining. I haven't found that to be the case. Yes, I have cancer, but it is not who I am. It's the seemingly little things (such as still having eyebrows when the rest of your hair is gone) that allow you to look in the mirror and still find yourself. Still feel like yourself. Having a terminal illness and feeling like myself—that's the freest I have ever felt.

Cancer didn't give this freedom to me.

I took it.

CHAPTER SEVEN

FEAR

Understanding Fear

Understanding fear can be a huge advantage. Throughout my personal and professional life, I have used inevitable fear to push me in the directions I needed to go.

All of us live with some measure of fear in our lives, no matter how courageous we think we might be. We are human. As children, we might have been afraid of thunderstorms or invisible monsters lurking under our bed. As teenagers, perhaps it was the fear of being uncool in school. Or flunking the driver's test. Or having to move to a new city and make a whole new set of friends.

As adults, the list becomes more complex and abstract: losing your job, becoming the victim of a violent crime, being diagnosed with a terminal illness. (Stage IV metastatic breast cancer comes immediately to mind.)

It's vital for us to understand the nature and origin of our fears, not just to understand the stuff that scares us but also to understand *why* this stuff scares us. Where does our fear come from? Coming to this understanding, arriving at this level of self-awareness, is the only way we can reach into ourselves and begin to unravel this mess that lives inside us.

Fear Isn't Failure

My awareness of fear allows me to channel it into something else. For as long as I can remember—long before my diagnosis—I've been able to transform my fear into a form of healthy, jet-propelled focus and then transform that focus into *action*.

As a goalie on the field hockey team, I was fiercely competitive, serious, and determined. While it was sometimes scary having the ball flying right at me, to be a great goalie, I had to jump toward the ball and not fear it. You don't sit back and wait for the ball to reach you. If you did that, it would end up in the net. You have to beat the ball to save it.

The obvious fear here is getting hit or hurt by the object trying to rush its way past you. However, that wasn't my fear. My fear was losing. In the same way, I don't fear the cancerous tumors in my breast. I fear the fact that if they spread beyond my breast, they could kill me. The ball coming toward me wasn't the risk; the risk was the ball getting past me.

Looking back on it now, I realize that I wasn't just diving toward the ball. I was also actively challenging the fear that, if I missed, the opposing team would score. So I'd get the ball out by any means necessary—kicking, blocking, and slide tackling.

I pounce on my fears when they come barreling toward me with overwhelming velocity. I reach up and knock them the hell out. I'm not saying I'm fearless. I'm saying that when fear does fill me up, I have to decide quickly what to do with it. I don't let my fear fester.

I am not afraid to be afraid. It gives me power. It gives me choices. It gives me freedom. Whether I'm hunkered down near the goalpost or facing the challenges of daily life, I've always had a healthy relationship with the things that scare me.

While my fear certainly is understandable, maybe even reasonable, I work hard to direct it toward a desired result rather than let it give me a reason to retreat. I often hear from friends how they fear getting scans or going to the doctor because they're afraid of what they might find. The majority of the time, they had nothing to fear. Going in for the scan or checkup actually wiped away their fears and reassured them that they were healthy. For the small percentage that do end up having something surface in those appointments, being equipped with that knowledge and data empowers them and their medical team to tackle it head-on.

In a very real way, I *need* my fear. I have learned how to make it work for me. I constantly choose to use my fear in my favor to push me toward what I want to accomplish. "Rolling with the punches" lowers the impact of the hit. Sometimes fear still gets a good punch in, but I have learned how to bounce back or redirect the punch entirely by redefining how I am going to use that fear to optimize my situation.

I'm not saying that I don't experience scary moments. Those moments come more than I'd like. I've noticed that what scares me most is not the cancer itself but how its steady progression will affect the quality of my life. But I've even learned to make this fear work in my favor by embracing each moment and cherishing every encounter as fully as I can.

My relationship with fear, then, actually *feeds* my superpower. My fear is a strength, not a weakness. I refuse to see my fear as failure. It is a necessary emotion as long as it's kept in check.

Embracing and transforming fear into something positive and actionable is not easy. However, it is very attainable and something I work hard at doing all the time. The checking of one's fear is definitely an inside job, and I've had more practice than I would have liked, so hopefully some of my examples can resonate.

If I receive not-so-great news about a lab result or a scan (more on scans later), I don't retreat to a corner and throw my head under the covers. I pick up the phone and start calling my doctors. I schedule follow-up appointments. I push and prod the receptionists and assistants to accelerate the timing on a test or an important follow-up visit. If I want to continue fighting this disease, I must make things happen. I cannot afford to let my fear immobilize me.

Paralysis, for me, is not an option; it's a death sentence. Not even terminal cancer will render me so frightened I cannot move. At all times and in every moment—no matter how depressed I become or even when I give my fear permission to settle into my heart and mind for a little longer than is comfortable—I remind myself that this cancer I carry within me is not a sign of failure or weakness on my part. It is just a disease.

I am a myriad of things, and not *one* of them is associated with failure! Even though my cancer has returned, which I definitely do not consider a personal failure on my part either but a medical reality, I know I must keep my fear in check. I don't have time to be messing around with uncontrolled fear.

Yes, it sucks that my cancer has spread, and I will beat it down with every ounce of strength I have within me, but I will also continue to live my life and embrace everything that comes my way because that's just the kind of person I am. But you don't need to be in the throes of a terminal illness to adopt this kind of can-do, "Fuck you, fear" mindset. The thing about steering your mind onto a different path is that anyone can do it.

Your Fear Is Not My Fear

I don't want to give the impression that I am fear*less* or that my inner courage and unflinching resolve are impenetrable. That's not the case at all.

It's just that I know how to stand in the solid center of this thing called fear. I have learned to strike a comfortable balance between toxic positivity and constant negativity. I flat-out refuse to live within either of those dangerous polarities, and I'm careful about hanging out with people who do. I'm just not interested in surrounding myself with people who are either blindingly positive or suffocatingly negative.

As a cancer patient, I am often forced to navigate the polarities of other people's fears. When well-meaning people tell me, "You're going to be just fine, and everything's going to be okay," they are channeling their own fears through me—or trying to, anyway. And I won't have it.

Terminal cancer and the prospect of death and dying are unsettling topics—and it's even more unsettling to be in the immediate proximity of someone who happens to be in the throes of the disease—but don't project fear onto the patient. We have got enough fear of our own to balance. We don't need yours, too.

I don't mean to sound heartless or ungrateful, but the **last thing** I want to hear from someone is the empty, vacuous assurance that everything's going to be okay and that I'm going "to beat" this thing because I'm so strong.

Where would I be if my medical team ascribed to this notion? Or if my closest friends and family members who are my fiercest advocates hid behind the emptiness of these words? And do these words mean that if I *don't* "beat this thing," I am weak, flawed, or a failure? No way. That's bullshit.

If you are frightened, find a productive way to deal with your fear. Don't assign others the task of making sure your sensibilities are soothed. This job belongs to you. *Your fear is not my fear.*

I want to share another example of how people can often (unwittingly) transpose their own fears onto others. For a person in cancer treatment, the decision to wear a wig or not wear a wig is totally and deeply personal. Before we lose our hair, we have the power to decide whether we are going to tell someone that we have cancer. Once we are bald, that conversation is decided for us. We are a stereotypical walking billboard for cancer. Whether to cover that up is a very personal and oftentimes heavy choice.

At different points in my cancer treatment, I've lost my hair as the result of chemo. During this time several well-meaning friends have either generously given me a wig that they think I'd like or suggested that I wear one to "accentuate the beauty of my face."

As grateful as I am for these seemingly magnanimous gestures, I am equally frustrated (and yes, resentful) of the irrational fear and ignorance that's at the root of them.

When someone suggests that I wear a wig while I'm in treatment, I feel like what they're *really* saying is, "Seeing you without hair makes me feel vulnerable, frightened, and uncomfortable. I don't like to be reminded of how sick you are or, worse yet, how sick I myself could one day become." They're uncomfortable—*frightened* is the more accurate word—at the sight of a bald woman.

I'm certainly not knocking anyone who decides to take the wig route. As I talked about with Jess, we all have different and valid reasons for what we choose, and I completely understand and respect all these unfair decisions we have to choose from. I've worn wigs myself, many times, when my mood is right, and my desire is there. While I sometimes like the way they looked for a photo op or a special event, I never quite felt like myself in them. Covering up my bald head didn't provide me comfort.

During periods when I don't have hair, when anyone makes the suggestion that I wear a wig or a head covering, I think, *Thanks, but no, thanks. I was not put on this earth to help you become more comfortable with the fact that I have cancer. I don't need to be reactive to your discomfort.*

That's the thing about fear: It's slippery and amorphous. It can take on different forms and disguises with such dexterity and sneakiness that you don't even know you feel it until you've said something stupid or done something unintentionally insensitive such as offering a bald friend the gift of a wig.

That's the very reason a gift registry for cancer patients is so important: Because it creates choices for patients to select whatever products will be most useful to them as they live their own lives. Patients know themselves best, and they deserve to decide what they need and what they want.

When you're selecting a gift for a friend who has just become a new mother, for instance, you don't force a brand of diapers or type of bottle on her. You usually go to the baby registry she's designed so that you can choose one of the gifts she's already decided she wants! So why shouldn't cancer patients be given this same optionality and choice by having their own registry?

Some Seriously Scary Stuff

In this chapter on fear, I think it would be contextual to list some of my own fears. For practical purposes, I'll also expand my definition of fear here. Not every item on the following list causes me heart-stopping, paralyzing fear. Some of these items are simply stress inducing, but since stress is a by-product of fear, I count it as fair game.

Facing My Own Fears

Needles

I've *always* been afraid of needles. I hate everything about them—how menacing they look lying on their antiseptic trays in the doctor's office or the lab. How patiently they wait for me, as if they're counting down the moments until they can get under my skin (literally). Their impossible pointiness.

How I manage my fear of needles: Most importantly, I understand the origin of my fear of needles. During my teenage and young adult years, I battled endometriosis, and injections were a regular and painful part of my reality. When I see a needle coming at me today, I remind myself that I dealt with them back then . . . and I can deal with them now. They are a known entity. I also remind myself that although the sight of the needle itself is menacing and super-scary the *function* of the needle—to deliver medicine into my body that helps preserve my life and keep my cancer in check—makes the power of its prick justifiable and necessary. Here's the long and short of it: *I need needles*, which mitigates my fear.

MRIs

I get a brain MRI about every nine weeks. In an MRI you are confined in a very tight space, with lots of clanging and loud noises. Picture a loud rave while lying in a casket. The funniest part is that I also always need an IV inserted for contrast, so I'm glad that we already addressed my fear of needles. It is imperative to remain *completely* motionless for the entire duration of the MRI (which, for me, can be anywhere from forty minutes to as long as two hours).

For my breast MRIs, I am laid out on a cold, flat slab of metal, on my stomach, with cutouts in the slab so that my breasts can protrude through the holes. A metal rod runs across the slab to stabilize and support my chest. It's uncomfortable and anxiety inducing on the best of days.

How I manage the discomfort and anxiety of MRIs: Each time I get an MRI, I channel thoughts of gratitude for the fact that I am not claustrophobic. I also whisper a silent shout-out to all the *children* who have to get MRIs, and while I'm trapped in that confined space, I often think about how very difficult it must be for them to lie totally motionless for such long periods. (Most children who have to get MRIs must receive anesthesia for this very reason.)

What also helps alleviate my discomfort with MRIs is when I remind myself that this procedure is not new to me. As an athlete who has sustained her fair share of sports injuries, I've also had my fair share of MRIs.

While these scans can be uncomfortable and scary, I would encourage you to embrace the importance of having the information necessary to stay on top of your health.

CT Scans

What I fear most about getting certain scans is that it might *miss something*. When the cancer recently returned in my left breast (for the third time), it was not the routine chest CT scan that picked it up; *it was the MRI that we ordered after the fact.* The breast scan actually came back clear, even though cancer was present.

Here's what's important: Even though the chest CT scan came back clear, I still felt like something was wrong; something within me felt similar to the way that my body felt when I was first diagnosed. My oncologist suggested that we look deeper into this sense of discomfort I was experiencing. She responded to my concerns, even after the scan came back clear, because I am so fortunate to have a medical team that addresses my concerns and doesn't dismiss them. She ordered the MRI, which revealed that the cancer had spread.

I am by no means pointing fingers or calling into question the overall efficacy of body scans—they are a lifesaving diagnostic, of that there is no question—but the fact of the matter is that different scans detect different things. I'm not angry that the CT scan didn't pick up the cancer; I'm grateful that the MRI did.

The biggest lesson that I've learned through these experiences of finding cancer in my body is that you have to utilize the tools available, but you also have to trust your instincts and intuition. If something doesn't feel right, the worst case is that you took the time to take a closer look. Utilizing scans and trusting your intuition of what feels right or wrong are not mutually exclusive ideas. You can do both, and I highly encourage you to utilize both.

These are examples of how I not only face and embrace my fears and anxieties but also choose to make them work in my favor.

If you don't do it, no one else will.

On Death and Dying

People generally aren't courageous enough to ask me, flat out, if I am afraid of dying—either because they're scared to hear my honest answer or because they're under the impression that by talking about the possibility/probability of someone else's death, they will hasten their own.

Just because people don't generally ask me about how I feel about dying, though, doesn't mean that I haven't pondered the question myself. I do have an answer, by the way, and the answer is this: I don't really think about death a whole hell of a lot.

Why? I am *far* more focused on the constant, ongoing process of living my life than on fearing my death.

As humans, we are all terminal; dying is as much a part of life as living is. As long as I am here and able to speak, to laugh, to cry, to help others, to raise my daughter, to love my husband, and to cherish my family and friends, I will choose to celebrate the living of my life rather than to mourn its inevitable final conclusion.

What I fear more than this cancer and even my eventual death, as I've mentioned before, is the prospect of no longer being able to determine or control the *quality* of my life. Sometimes these thoughts put me in a dark place, and I allow myself to stand in this darkness for a time, because it, too, is a legitimate place within which to stand: I just refuse to stay stuck there.

When I speak this bluntly about death, I am often told, "Careful, don't put that out into the universe." They warn me not to manifest or talk about it because then it might come true. I choose to embrace the fact that I will eventually die because it empowers me to take back control over the time I have. None of us know how much time that is, with or without cancer.

I am not saying that I'm dying anytime soon; I am saying that someday I will die. We all will die someday. This is an inevitable truth for all of us. We all have risks in our life and at any moment could meet a tragic end. I am constantly reminded by people that any of us could have a sudden heart attack or get in a car wreck.

I cannot control or predict the moment I will die—none of us can—but I *can* control how much mental energy I give to worrying about it.

As the founder of a nonprofit devoted to helping people in the cancer community, however, the statistical reality is that I lose more friends to cancer because I *have* more friends with cancer. I have no regrets about living within this stark statistic, either. I regret that my friends die, certainly, but I do not regret that they lived. This helps me embrace my grief in a healthy way because it helps me understand that grief is born out of love. I am grateful for that love.

My circumstances, then, have taught me how to stand in the middle of grief *and* gratitude. It's the healthiest place to be because it allows me to celebrate the wins and to mourn the losses at the same time.

The people I have loved and lost have had a positive impact on my life and on this world in a way that endures. That remains alive and vibrant long after they themselves have taken their last breath.

This is why my work with WeGotThis.org is so important to me. The contributions people make to the organization (not just financial, of course, but also time, energy, and love) have an impact that lasts. That's how I see love itself: infinite and immutable. It endures forever. I know that I am very fortunate to have developed this sensibility and heightened awareness, and I will carry it with me always.

I recently traveled to Boston for WeGotThis.org. I'd just come back from New York City for the same reasons, and these trips required a tremendous amount of my energy, but I was happy to do them because it helped move our nonprofit forward.

Boston was successful on many levels. While I was there, I had a chance to meet a new friend who was in treatment for colon cancer. She coincidentally finished chemo the day that I arrived, so we went to surprise her and her family to celebrate.

Only hours after I celebrated the end of my friend's chemo, though, I received the news that another friend (in California) had just succumbed to colon cancer.

She was a mom, just like me. In fact, I met her because her daughter was in Ellie's preschool class. I suffer from survivor's guilt—why is her daughter now without a mother and Ellie is fortunate enough to still have me close?—and I'm also really pissed off at this ravaging, indiscriminate disease.

As I've already said, nobody "loses their battle" with cancer. I believe that they fight it for as long as they possibly can. She was a winner, and while I certainly count her death as a loss (in the most literal sense because the world has lost her), *I count her life as a win*—a huge win.

This is how I choose to embrace this concept of death and dying—not by being immobilized with grief when people I know pass away but by being propelled and fortified by the positive impact these people had on the world and on me specifically.

If I focus only on the loss—only on death—then I am giving the disease of cancer far too much power. I will not look at cancer—my own or anyone else's—as just a death sentence. I am more than my own eventual death.

You are more than your eventual death, too.

Let's focus on the things we can control and what we know we can control in this minute. This moment, right now, in front of us.

In these moments, let's choose to live.

CHAPTER EIGHT

CHILDREN

The Best Parent for Your Child Is You

Shortly after our daughter was born, I remember having a conversation with a dear friend of mine about parenting. At the time Eric and I were juggling new parenthood *and* my recent cancer diagnosis, so a lot of things were swirling around us.

Normally I'm a little leery of people who offer parenting advice, only because the process of parenting is so deeply personal. However, because this friend is someone I respect, I knew his advice was coming from a good place. I decided it was worth my time to hear him out, and I am so glad that I did.

He said (and I'm obviously paraphrasing):

> When you have your daughter, all of the advice everyone throws at you will feel overwhelming. If there's anything I've learned from being the dad of two daughters, it's that nobody could ever be better parents to them than my wife and I. No matter what we do, it's the right thing because it's us, and that's how it will be for both of you. You and Eric will know your child better than anyone else in the world. This is the only thing

that truly matters. Most of the other unsolicited advice is just noise.

In that moment it really did feel like he was handing me the gift of his simple wisdom that I could pick up and possess as my own. All the inner strength and innate wisdom that I needed as a parent already rested within me.

Particularly as a new parent, or as a parent grappling with a life challenge that might adversely affect your entire family, advice from others is going to come flying at you from all directions. Trust me on this.

But whether you take that advice is up to you.

This universal truth automatically makes us members of the same club. While each of our parenting principles is obviously unique—you've got yours and I've got mine—it sure feels good to be able to share wisdom and encouragement between us. When it comes to walking with your children through a difficult moment or a trying time, you're stronger than you think you are.

Communication Is Key

How you communicate and interact with your child is your personal decision; it's a decision that belongs to no one else but you.

There is no single way of living or a specific way of being. Each person's life is different and beautifully unique; what works in my life will not necessarily work in yours, but I hope some of my experiences resonate in your life as well.

I have always spoken openly and honestly with my daughter about the fact that I have cancer. It's not our *only* topic of conversations, thank goodness, because cancer is not the only thing I focus on in my daily life. I flat-out refuse to allow it to take up all our emotional space. But I owe it to my daughter and to myself to approach this topic with respect and honesty.

As a parent, I see it as my responsibility and my absolute joy to celebrate the beautiful wholeness of life with my daughter. I want her to see and feel the different textures that each day brings, the smooth surfaces and the bumpy, rocky places that are sometimes difficult to navigate.

Eric and I want Ellie, even as young as she is, to have a vision that's as big as ours are. *Nothing about us is narrow.* Life is full of color. Sometimes those colors get a little dark and daunting, but we're always authentic, honest, and open about how we approach those dark spots, too. When we talk with her, we want her to know that what she's feeling and experiencing is valid: the bright and colorful, the gray and dreary, and every rainbow mix in between!

As she gets older and becomes more able to process and understand the complexities of cancer, we'll talk with her about the topic on a more intellectual level. But for now we are precisely where we need to be. My daughter knows I have cancer, but she also knows that yesterday we made cookies, and tonight we're going to dance in our kitchen.

My cancer for her then is contextual. We explore the topic when it becomes contextually relevant for us to explore it—when

I've lost (or cut) my hair, for instance, or when I'm not feeling all that great and would rather stay in bed for a few extra hours.

Always, though, our communication comes from a gentle, loving place that confronts our reality but doesn't linger in a dark, frightening place. Frightening places are not good for anybody. That is not where I am, and it is not where we want our daughter to be.

Every parent has to navigate, at some point or another, how best to communicate with their child when the waves get rough and the waters get deep. If you are grappling with a challenge in your life that's difficult or daunting to discuss with your own children, just know you are not the first. Remind yourself of this when you feel most isolated. **You are not alone.**

Living with a terminal disease requires far more than just the desire and the willingness to communicate with my daughter freely and openly. The words are important, but what's more important are my **acts.** *It is vital that Ellie sees her mommy living her life. Doing her thing. Pushing out into the world every day without fear. Helping others who are on this same road. Shining my light, making a difference, and leaving my fingerprint on the world.*

Ellie needs to see me embracing each day with purpose and passion. Living boldly and without apology. Nurturing friendships. Raising awareness (and funding) for my nonprofit that helps others living with cancer. Being a loving wife and a supercool mom. Being bald (when necessary). Throwing up (when necessary) and kicking cancer's ass, thank you very much. She needs to see me making pancakes with her on Saturday morning and dancing together to Backstreet Boys and NSYNC! (Yes, we love *both* of them.)

I communicate not only with my words but also with my actions.

"Bless You, Mommy!"

I felt severely nauseous during chemo and was confined to bed for ten to fourteen days at a time every three weeks. I didn't like the fact that being bedridden reduced the precious time I spent with my little girl, so I made adjustments whenever I could.

Some mornings, when I was too sick to get out of bed, Eric would bring her into our bed for a warm snuggle and some precious mommy-daughter time. Other times I'd *force* myself out of bed, not just to hang out with my daughter in another part of the house but also to assert a degree of control over my own condition.

I remember one particular *force-yourself-out-of-bed* morning. I was determined to walk my husband and my daughter to the front door for a proper goodbye before they left for the day, but my rising nausea said, "Not today."

I never made it to the front door.

Hell, I barely made it to the bathroom.

Ellie had certainly heard me throw up before, but I just wanted to create *one precious, puke-free morning* for her so she wouldn't associate her mommy with only being sick. I could hear her little feet running toward the bathroom door.

Please don't open that door, babe, I thought. *Seeing Mommy barfing her brains out is not the way I want you to start your day.*

I mean, there is a limit to the sights and sounds I want to share with my daughter as I endure this crappy condition. As parents, we have to know our children well enough to decide the amount of information that's right to share with them, particularly in the midst of an unpleasant situation or an ongoing crisis. It's up to us to decide how much information is enough information—and when it is too much.

My sweet girl didn't open the door, thank goodness, but she did holler out one of the sweetest affirmations of pure love I've ever heard:

"Bless you, Mommy!"

She thought I was *sneezing* (not vomiting), and she was simply being polite and compassionate! Hearing her "bless me" with such purity and innocence made me smile, and it made me feel so deeply loved, even while I was down on my knees throwing up.

Here I was, so worried that she'd be upset or frightened, but it turned out I was only projecting my own adult fears onto her. When I opened that bathroom door and saw her beautiful little face, I realized she wasn't worried at all. She was only saying what polite people *say* when they hear someone else sneeze: "Bless you!"

In that moment she definitely blessed me, all right, and I will never forget it.

Living with cancer doesn't easily lend itself to balance, but I am very proud of the way Eric and I have established important, appropriate balances and boundaries with our daughter around this disease while also being as open, honest, and age appropriate as we possibly can.

As much as I love living life, I will be the first to admit that raising a child while living with a terminal illness can be turbulent at times. But I embrace the turbulence with every ounce of strength I have within me; I owe it to my daughter, to my husband, and to myself. Every second I spend with them is precious.

For this reason, I work hard to make sure that my *relationship* with Ellie—as well as Ellie's understanding of cancer itself—is balanced and realistic. I do not want her to only associate cancer with death and dying; it has to be more than that.

I want her to associate cancer with life and living as well! My daughter needs to understand that, yes, her mother happens to have cancer, but this disease is not the sole factor that defines her life. I live my life fully, and I am proud of the way I have shown her how I live with cancer.

I take great pride in the fact that our daughter sees both her mother and her father living their very best lives, doing the things that they love most in the world. Even at her young age, she knows, deep down in that little heart of hers, that she is so incredibly loved.

So many things in the world are uncontrollable, but this is not one of them. My daughter knows that she is cherished beyond measure. I am certain she knows it.

I would stake my life on it.

A Home to Hold Us

There were some days, early on, when I simply could not function. Eric showered me with comfort—enough to cover both me and our daughter—and even my mother would come to stay with us for weeks at a time.

Around this time was when we considered the possibility of moving into a new home, a bigger, more accommodating place that had a guesthouse for when we needed the additional help of a visiting family member.

We didn't just see this as a pipe dream. This was a medical and emotional necessity that had the potential of enhancing the quality of our lives tremendously, provided we could find the right home.

As always, Eric and I were methodical in our approach. While Eric began researching different possibilities, I started making calls and exploring next steps. I called my accountant and my financial advisor—and I put my own financial management cap on again. We needed to be able to make a finite assessment about whether this was a distant dream or an attainable reality.

Evaluating whether to make the biggest purchase of our lives required a lot of number crunching, meticulous evaluation, family discussions, and plenty of research. I've always worked incredibly fast because there's no time like the present, and I certainly have no time to waste! In this case it took a couple of weeks to find the home of our dreams—a place of peace, comfort, and calm that was everything we could ask for and more.

The home had a separate guesthouse for relatives who would be visiting to help on those days when I couldn't really function. It had cozy bedrooms, a sunlight-filled living room, and enough space for us to create a small playground for Ellie, especially useful when I didn't feel well enough to take her to a public park or to the community playground. We were looking for a home that could suit our specific needs. A home that could be our haven.

When I asked my therapist what she thought about this potentially major move, her response was straightforward, as always: "The house sounds like it's perfectly suited for your family, Elissa. *Your home should hold you.*"

That's precisely what our home does: Our home holds us.

We have fundraisers right here in our backyard. Ellie has her own bedroom filled with her own furniture. (Okay, so it's the furniture that I won when I was a contestant on the TV show *Let's Make a Deal*, but it belongs to Ellie now, and she definitely claims it as her own!)

She has a home that *holds* her today, and this same home will hold her tomorrow, the year after that, and the year after that and as we create new memories moving forward. She was potty trained in her own little bathroom—if that's not a "life marker," then I don't know what is! She's developing her own sense of style, distinct tastes, and unique preferences. Her closet only holds clothes that she likes and that she has selected herself. (Gone are the days when Mommy picks out her clothes!) She dresses up for the fundraising events we have here at our home, and she thoroughly enjoys being the belle of the ball.

Were we taking a risk in moving forward with this purchase? You bet we were—a young child, unknown medical expenses, questions about my own future. But it was a careful, calculated risk, and we embraced the fact that sometimes doing the right thing for your family might sometimes mean moving beyond your comfort zone, stepping into unknown waters, and pushing out into new territory.

We Love Ourselves Some Lemons!

As I've mentioned, having a guesthouse was very important to us, and we were willing to tighten our belts and make the necessary sacrifices to get it. When you're faced with a chronic condition or a terminal illness, having a place where people can hunker down close by for extended periods is crucial. Creating such an accommodation is not always possible, which is why we feel particularly fortunate to have been able to make this dream a reality.

When my mom visits, sometimes for weeks at a time, the guesthouse provides a dedicated, stand-alone space for her. Knowing that she's only steps away also provides tremendous emotional security. From a medical perspective, I can say without hesitation that my mother's proximity is *healing*.

Shortly after we moved into our new home, my mom expressed an interest in planting a lemon tree just outside the guesthouse. Was the idea of being able to literally live out the saying "When life gives you lemons . . ." a bit on the nose? Admittedly yes, but I always lean into a good corny joke.

Our little lemon tree began producing lemons almost immediately—big, *healthy* lemons, too! Each time I look at our lemon tree (which is every day), it makes me grin to think about our family's decision to not dwell on life's lemons but to embrace them and grow our own.

You don't have to wait for life to give you lemons. Grow your own damn lemons and make whatever you want with them.

Find Your Inner Child

My dear friend, singer-songwriter, creative coach, keynote speaker, award-winning podcast host, and executive producer Lauren LoGrasso totally changed my life when she shared with me her knowledge and wisdom surrounding the subject of childhood and creativity. I invited her to share the same with you here.

Notes on Creativity

Creativity is often seen as a luxury—a pursuit for those with time, talent, or the right circumstances. But what if I told you that creativity is not a privilege but rather a birthright that we all have the power to reclaim? Believe it, baby!

Elissa and I first met when she was a guest on my podcast back in 2021, and at that time, believe it or not, she didn't consider herself creative. She felt this even though she was literally doing something no one had ever done before in creating WeGotThis.org. But sadly, this belief about lacking creativity is more common than you'd think. Throughout the years, we somehow detach from this deep part of life and who we are . . . But why? And how?

It doesn't start out this way. On the contrary, as little kids, creativity was part of pretty much everything we did. From dress up to painting to singing and make-believe, it ran through everything. So what happened?

Well, according to a longitudinal study conducted by NASA, it was very visibly knocked out of us and by a villain you wouldn't necessarily expect. This study followed a ground of 1,600 children from the ages of five up until they were thirty-one, and the results were stunning and heartbreaking.

At age five, 98 percent of children score at a "creative genius" level. However, by age ten, then genius tag dropped to 30 percent, and by fifteen it is was down to 12 percent. By the end of the study, at thirty-one, only a dismal 2 percent maintained the level of creative genius.

So what was the monster sucking out all the creativity? According to the study, our creativity is drained by our education. As we learn to excel at convergent thinking—or the ability to focus and hone our thoughts—we squash our instinct for divergent or generative thought, a.k.a. daydreaming and creative flow. We also learn there are consequences to "being wrong," and that creates all kinds of negative ripples over what we think we're capable of and/or willing to share.

But here's the good news from this: You were born a creative genius, and therefore, creativity isn't something you have to invent or conjure up but rather just remember.

So what can you do today? The first step is getting back in touch with your inner child. Ask yourself what you loved to do as a child. What did you love to do before anyone told you to be practical? (Or that you weren't good enough or that you were wrong.) What did little you just purely love? Then start doing that. In low-pressure situations, start incorporating it in. Journal about it, visualize it, start practicing, share it with someone . . .

And the next thing to do is ask yourself this: If you found out you had limited time on this earth, what would you want to spend time doing? Elissa so poignantly reminds us: We DO have limited time—no matter what your current level of health, we're all terminal. And truthfully I find that inspiring. It's our greatest call to action to live.

So today I ask you to remember the beginning (your inner child) and remember the end (our mortality) so you can fully live in the present and have the courage to be yourself. Unleash your inner creative, find your authentic voice, and gain the courage to pursue all of your wildest dreams.

CHAPTER NINE

CAREGIVING

The Invisible Patient

When I turned eighteen, I went skydiving for the first time with some high school friends. When you jump out of a plane, you have to remain calm. When you're in that free fall, panicking is simply not an option. If you do panic, you can't breathe. *You must stay calm.* There are powerful parallels between falling through the sky and falling into the role of cancer patient that I did not ask for and did not see coming.

I always aim to create calm in the midst of crisis; it gives me the space I need to figure out my next steps and strategize my plan of attack. In this case remaining calm and lucid also allowed me to absorb and process everything the oncologist was telling me in real time. I had to remain cool and calm while I was falling through *that* sky; paralyzing fear was not an option.

Looking back on both of those experiences—diving from that plane and sitting in that doctor's office—I could easily have lost my breath . . . but I didn't. This fills me with a sense of pride, gratitude, and wonder: When calm is required, I create it. My life depends on it.

Sitting in that oncologist's office was very much like literally falling through the sky. Every instinct told me to hold my breath or cry hot tears or holler for help, but in both instances, I was able to relax my mind and body. Because, of course, I didn't just have a sense of calm; *I also had a parachute.*

As I was falling through those clouds, you better believe I pulled the *hell* out of that rip cord and came to a safe landing (even though I threw up as soon as I landed). At the oncologist's, my parachute happened to be sitting right beside me, the man who would become the best caregiver a person could ever ask for: my husband, Eric.

Our caregivers are our parachutes. They keep us afloat and alive. They ensure our "safe landing" each and every day. If they weren't in our lives, we'd certainly be in a free fall.

We wouldn't have chosen "caregiver" for one of Eric's titles at this stage of life, but I am grateful that he has embraced it the way he has. This is how I look at it: If I have to have cancer, who better a caregiver to have on my side and in my life than the man of my dreams? Who better to have in my corner than this human being who not only brings me joy and comfort but also my *meds*?

Navigating the wild world of medications, particularly for someone with a chronic or terminal illness, can be daunting for both the patient *and* the caregiver. It almost feels like you're a mouse in a maze, scurrying this way and that, trying to keep up with all the twists, turns, and unexpected detours—the constantly changing dosages, the possibility of negative side effects, or the dangerous potential of an allergic reaction or some other unanticipated hiccup.

Some of my meds must be taken on an empty stomach, others on a full stomach. Some must be taken in the morning, others in the afternoon. Or late afternoon. Or bedtime. Or just before bedtime.

Certain meds must be stored at room temperature. Others must be refrigerated. A few of my meds need to be stopped a specific number of days before chemo begins, then others must be taken for a specific number of days *after* chemo. (And I should add, some pills are actually chemo treatments!)

When I first started treatment, I had to give myself injections for a certain number of consecutive days after the infusion to protect my bones. While I hate needles, I wanted to do it myself to feel in control. I would hype myself up before each injection, like getting ready to leap out of that plane. After each shot was a big sigh of relief and a proud moment that I was tough enough to finish the job.

Then there are the prescriptions I must have on hand at all times for special toothpastes and mouth rinses to stay ahead of the cold sores that can often develop during chemo. The list is endless. Eric keeps the process meticulously organized, the prescriptions current, the dosages accurate, the train on track. If I happen to be away from home when it's time to take a specific medicine, he'll always text me with a reminder: "It's time!"

This kind of constant vigilance represents only a small slice of what Eric does for me. Do I sometimes get annoyed when someone is always checking in to make sure I took my meds? Yes, I do. But I love him for it, and I know that each dose of keeping my cancer under control is medicine for the both of us.

In a very real way, I owe my life (as well as the *quality* of my life) to Eric. He is my constant supporter. Even though he has his own life, his own career, his own passions, and his own interests, he always knows how and when to "combine" his energy with mine when it's necessary. When it comes to relating to my husband as my primary caregiver, I also try to make the intentional effort to understand and appreciate what it must feel like to be in *his* shoes. What does he encounter each and every day? What does *he* think about in those moments when he is caring for his wife or on daddy/daughter duty because I'm too sick to help out? How often does he have to picture the nightmare of me not being there with them anymore? His perspective *matters*. His needs *matter*.

We are usually so focused on the visceral and immediate needs, desires, and concerns of the *patient* that we completely overlook the needs, desires, and concerns of the *caregiver*. This imbalance can create deep fissures and friction, both mental and physical, and often contributes to some of the things that caregivers struggle with, such as extreme anxiety, depression, fear, isolation, and hopelessness.

The parachute doesn't get a big round of applause when it lands safely to the ground. Nobody praises the parachute for a safe landing. The parachute is a key player in this equation, but it is always overlooked and ignored. If it works, we don't pay it any attention.

This is why the caregiver is so often referred to as "the invisible patient." They are rarely seen or heard, yet they, too, are in need of care and attention. There's no doubt that these heroes deserve a voice. They deserve to be heard.

I have invited my husband, Eric, to share his perspective. His words are worthy of attention; his viewpoint holds value. So here, I yield the floor—and the page—to him.

How It Feels

Within the year leading up to Elissa's cancer diagnosis, our family went through many changes. Our daughter, Ellie, was born in the middle of the pandemic, we drove across the country twice with a two-month-old so she could meet her extended family, we moved into a new house, and we started a four-month renovation of our kitchen and bathrooms. The day before the diagnosis, we were deep in the renovations and anxiously waiting for results from the biopsy. If it wasn't for me randomly touching my wife while she was changing in our closet, I would have never felt the growth in her breast, and we would never have known that she had breast cancer.

I remember exactly where we were when she told me. Elissa walked into my office and revealed the results, and I started tearing up. As a couple, we had been through many tough times over the years between my mother having stage IV non-Hodgkin's lymphoma, Elissa's brother passing away at the young age of thirty-one, and Elissa having a miscarriage a year earlier. I knew we were tough and could handle hard things, but never did I think we would have something like this so early on in our journey as new parents.

Our daughter was about to turn a year old in mere days, and my mind immediately went to the dreaded "what-ifs."

- What if we only have days/weeks/months with Elissa?
- What if Ellie never gets to know her mother?
- What if I become a single dad with a toddler?

For a couple of weeks, I cried every day, consumed by this cloud of dread. It got worse when I hyperventilated/nearly passed out when I saw the PET scan show that the cancer spread all around her liver and lymph nodes. Elissa is very good at holding her emotions together, but I always have been known to wear my heart on my sleeve.

Before we knew it was stage IV, we were under the impression that this would be cured. However, Elissa started to understand that this was going to be a forever battle, and she needed me to also face the reality. It was during this time that I started to add the biggest "hat" to my collection of multitasking hats: husband, father, son, brother, musician, runner, and now, caretaker.

It was really hard to adjust to this role. There was a lot of note-taking at appointments, alarms I set on my phone for medications, food that I prepped for my wife and daughter, and many times of being alone with my thoughts. I luckily had the help of my mother-in-law (who happened to be in town at the time) to switch back and forth with me between caring for Elissa and Ellie, but there were a couple of things I wish I could have told myself back then:

1. Take care of yourself so you can take care of others.
2. When people offer help, take it.

I put myself last on my priority list, and it showed. I wasn't playing music, I would only go for a run once in a while, and I was very depressed. I would have to leave the house with Ellie and go to a park or a store just to get away from the big emotions that were always there. There were times I would cry in the car for a good five to ten minutes, releasing all the energy I had been feeling. One time I was in the car holding and hugging a sixteen-month-old Ellie, and I swear that she consciously rubbed my back to tell me that "It was okay." I held on tight to this beautiful little girl, as she was my saving grace through all this.

I was also having a hard time allowing for help and finding people who were in the same boat as me. I thought that taking pride in being the "sole caretaker" meant that I had to do everything myself, but that's not true at all. It's foolish to think that anyone could juggle all these responsibilities alone. I slowly started building a team that could help us, and I wish I had done it sooner.

The first year of caretaking was hard. The second year was even tougher as Elissa battled brain tumors, a recurrence, and medical trials that left her bedridden. The third year has been easier than the previous years, but it will always have its challenges. By now I have grown some really thick skin. I can take on a lot more than I ever thought I could. I've compared the handling of hard things to lifting a heavy dumbbell: I've lifted it so many times that it feels easy now.

I also have come to the philosophy that caretaking is like the weather: Sometimes a sunny-day forecast will bring unexpected rain. When that happens, you have no choice but to pivot.

Therapy was one of the ways I started taking care of myself, and a therapist had me answer the same "what-if" questions that I asked myself during Elissa's initial diagnosis. This time I had to answer the questions realistically. As we went through each one, it gave me some solace to have a "plan" of sorts if it ever happened. By doing the exercise, I didn't have to dread it anymore. It helped me understand that asking "what-if" creates too many expectations and fears versus saying, "This is the reality, and this is how I will handle it."

Being a caretaker has shown me more than ever that I don't have time to sweat the small things. I have a responsibility to take care of the two most important people in my life while also taking care of myself. I ask for help when I absolutely need it (still working on that). When we get tough news or Elissa doesn't feel well, I pivot and understand what I have to do next. I am proud of the man I've become during the tough times, and I will continue to grow this caretaker armor in the years to come.

If you are living with a chronic condition and are fortunate enough to have someone offering you care and support on a regular basis and in a loving, attentive manner, consider reaching out to them and asking them to share their personal perspective. Reading Eric's experience gave me insight deeper than what I think he could have expressed to me in person. We all have a cancer story; they're just not all from the perspective of the patient.

Dr. Jamie Jacobs, the head of the caregivers research program for Massachusetts General Brigham in Boston, is a noted authority and respected voice on caring for caregivers. At this writing, WeGotThis.org is working with Dr. Jacobs to fund their young adult caregivers research at the hospital, which is vital and necessary research for the wider cancer community. (Jacobs is, in fact, on the board of directors of WeGotThis.org and provides invaluable guidance and insight as we continue to interface with this vital and growing segment of the population.)

Here, she offers her insights on caregivers, particularly for the adolescent and young adult population in the cancer community.

Caring for the Caregiver

Caregivers are an integral member of the oncology team, often tasked with providing care, ensuring medication adherence, and managing symptoms, particularly as more medical care is delivered in the outpatient setting or at home, and hospital stays become shorter. They are thrust into these roles with little information or preparedness and without much choice in the matter. Caregivers often selflessly give their time to caring, supporting administering medications, driving to and from medical appointments and procedures, while managing their own jobs and other dependent family members and children. We hear directly from caregivers how they are stretched thin with little time to spare for themselves. It is no wonder we are learning that caregivers are experiencing more physical ailments from colds to heart disease, as well as mood disorders like depression and anxiety. Caregivers are worn out and at growing risk for serious chronic illness and mortality themselves.

Learning practical skills to cope with distress can have a major influence on a family caregiver's quality of life. We are in the process of testing several therapeutic programs based in cognitive behavioral therapy, mindfulness-based cognitive therapy, acceptance commitment therapy, and relaxation training. Some of these programs are for the caregiver alone, while others put the patient and caregiver together with a therapist. The therapists focus on delivering practical, concrete skills for coping with stress, having meaningful conversations, managing physical and emotional symptoms with behavioral techniques, and helping caregivers find ways to prioritize self-care. We have already show some promising results, and are committed to improving the lives of cancer caregivers.

We are working to help you, the caregiver. Our goal is to keep moving forward so that one day these programs will be incorporated into the clinical care that we deliver. Personally, my goal is for every caregiver who walks through the door to be able to access supportive care services. Caregivers all over should have the opportunity to receive the type of support that helps them. Caregivers deserve their own support systems and to prioritize their own self-care, both for their own benefit and the benefit of the person with cancer. You are not invisible.

Yay for AYA!

We've already lamented the caregiver (in many cases) as "the invisible patient." But there's also another group within the cancer community that often goes unseen and unheard as well: the adolescent and young adult (AYA) sector of the population.

The National Comprehensive Cancer Network guidelines define an AYA oncology patient as **an individual between fifteen and thirty-nine years of age** at the time of the initial diagnosis.

Sadly, the number of young adults living with this disease is on the rise, which also means that the number of caregivers in the AYA community is rising.

I was thirty-four at the time of my diagnosis, and am thirty-seven now, so I can certainly and directly relate. Members of the AYA cancer community face a unique and complicated set of circumstances. I mean, it's wild to think that if I were pregnant right now, I would be considered a geriatric pregnancy, the category used to describe women who are pregnant at thirty-five and older, but having cancer right now makes me a young adult. I'll take the wins where I can get them, I guess?

What are normally the pivotal, life-defining "markers" in any young person's life—landing that first job, launching a career, finding a spouse, starting a family—become potential snares when you have to navigate these important life transitions with cancer.

I'm not saying these pivotal life markers become any less exciting, but the presence of cancer (or any chronic or terminal illness, for that matter) creates an entirely new layer of detours. In the same way that we need to see, hear, and value the views and perspectives of our caregivers, we need to give equal space and grace to our young people who are living with the disease. To overlook them—even if we overlook them unintentionally—is insensitive and irresponsible. We need to do better, to open our eyes wider so that our vision includes this forgotten demographic as well.

WeGotThis.org works very closely with hospitals, as you might imagine, and the good news is that a growing number of hospitals seem to be bringing on AYA coordinators: dedicated staff who focus on the specific needs of this growing population. But unfortunately, overall progress in this area is slow, and the disparity remains significant.

We plan to change this trend.

Dr. Marla Lipsyc-Sharf, breast medical oncologist, is a leading authority on metastatic breast cancer, and I'm proud to say that she's my oncologist! I hold Dr. Sharf in the highest regard, not only because of her impeccable credentials and reputation but also for the invaluable wisdom and guidance she has shared with me personally throughout my cancer journey.

She said, "Young adults with breast cancer are often dealing with a unique set of challenges. As they undergo treatment for breast cancer, they may also be managing families, careers, social lives, dating, education, and other pursuits. As an oncologist, it is clear to me that all of my patients are individuals with different values and priorities. I am grateful when patients share these priorities with me so that, together, we can pursue treatments that take these priorities into account."

Though progress is slowly being made on this front, those in the AYA community deserve a dedicated space of their *own*. The fact that cancer patients in this particular group—which, again, includes me—fall between the cracks is both harrowing and heartbreaking.

I know patients in their *twenties* who sit beside eight-year-olds in the waiting room of the pediatric oncologist who is treating them all. We have hospitals that are devoted exclusively to children. We have hospitals that are dedicated exclusively to adults. AYAs are in need of their own "home."

It's time to recognize that we are too large a group to be glossed over and overlooked any longer. We hear all the time that we're "too young to have cancer," but statistically, we are anything but. I literally cannot count all the friends I have who have cancer.

WeGotThis.org is vitally aware of this growing population, and we work hard to ensure that AYAs feel like they have a space and a place within our community.

While I'm a member of that community, I wanted to make space for another to share her story. Lisa Orr, a breast cancer survivor herself, is a masterclass in creating spaces for others to share their stories. She's the brand director of *Elephants and Tea*, a magazine written by and for the AYA cancer community. I've contributed in the past and felt it only right to have her contribute here.

The Reality of Being an "AYA": Entering the Unseen Bubble

I didn't know what the term "AYA" meant until I was one.

Unfortunately, I think that's a common reality of people that are handed a cancer diagnosis at a young age and are forced to join this "club" that none of us want to be a part of.

AYA stands for "adolescent and young adult," and it represents a community within the oncology space that is special for a lot of reasons . . . and no, I'm not using special in a positive way here. We are unique in that facing a cancer diagnosis at our age is less common and comes with a hell of a lot more challenges than older individuals may face when given a similar diagnosis.

Adolescents and young adults are supposed to be in their "prime." The great big world is out there, and they are ready to go out and make something of themselves. They are just beginning to figure out what career may fill their cups, they are in their key years of forming various types of relationships that will hopefully last decades to come, and they are, most of the time, doing all of this while living paycheck to paycheck.

Young adults are just beginning to learn how to navigate the ever-changing and increasingly tricky health-care system even as health individuals. Many are just coming off of their parents' insurance, forgetting to make their yearly checkup appointments, and honestly are just trying to survive the day-to-day hustle and bustle that our society promotes. Young people are often known to ignore aches and pains or chalk them up to a whole slew of believable ailments that they may face on a regular basis.

But then they do notice something that lingers. They gain the courage to ask a friend or family member about it, and they take the time to make an appointment or speak to a health-care professional about this ongoing symptom. They are learning to be more independent and confident, so you can understand their frustration when they are often told, "Oh, it's probably nothing. Maybe it's just [filling in the blank with any number of 'normal' nonserious health issues they could be facing]." So they go about their lives, trusting the advice of the older professional in the white coat because that is what they have done for their entire existence. Until . . . the symptom doesn't go away. It, in fact, gets worse, or changes, and now they are forced to speak up for themselves—a skill that is quite difficult to learn.

They may feel silly approaching their health-care team yet again with the same complaints. They may be faced with more excuses, more hesitation from the professionals, but the best-case scenario is that deep down they know something is wrong, so they keep advocating for themselves.

Navigating the uncertainties of life as a young adult can be difficult enough as it is, and then *boom*, along comes the dreaded cancer diagnosis that *no one* saw coming. Whether you've had older relatives with cancer, or you have been lucky enough to not have cancer touch your life up until this point, it is now your unfortunate reality. One day your most difficult decision is figuring out what to eat for dinner, and the next it's what treatment options are available to you and will I lose my job and can I still have kids and who will help support me and the list goes on and on and on . . .

For me, one of the hardest parts of my diagnosis was the sheer overload of information a young adult is handed within those first few days and weeks. It was the complete shock that I felt when the radiologist uttered the words "breast cancer" to me over the phone. It was the waterfall of questions and the "you are so brave," and it was the deep, terrifying feeling of being alone.

I was lucky to have an incredible support system of family and friends. I know that this is sadly not the case for everyone.

When I say I felt alone, I mean that I didn't know of anyone who had been diagnosed around my age. It is an incredibly lonely feeling knowing you are going through something so difficult with no guidance or support from someone who truly understands what you are going through. It wasn't until my sister stumbled upon a website that was a space for adolescent and young adult patients, survivors, and caregivers to share the stories of what they were going through that I knew there were others out there like me. And as it turns out, there's a lot of us.

The AYA cancer community is often referred to as a "bubble." Once you have entered the bubble, you see how many of us there actually are, all working toward the common goals of staying alive and supporting each other through the ups and downs of our cancer experiences. It became evidently clear to me that unless you were in that bubble, you didn't know it existed. Want to hear something crazy? The bubble even exists in the health-care system. I bet that if you were to approach ten different oncologists from ten different cities, maybe only about half of them (if that) would recognize the term "AYA."

The good news? There are so many amazing people and organizations that are working hard every single day to continue to spread the awareness and the realities of what life with cancer as a young adult is like. I feel beyond lucky to now be the brand director for one of them. There is so much power in community. I truly believe that human connection is what this world survives on, and knowing the hard work that is being done to not only create safe spaces for AYAs to find community but also to work toward spreading knowledge and resources for all who hear throw dreaded words makes me feel like the generations of AYAs to come will be in a better spot than even I was.

If it weren't for the AYAs whom I connected with, who helped guide me through the process and showed me that there was hope and that I wasn't alone in all that I was feeling and experiencing, I don't know if I would have the strength today to do the same for those who have come after me. I couldn't be happier that I picked up Elissa's phone call that day. That I was able to be an ear for her, to let her know that even on the other side of the country, she had a friend who understood. To see her not only answer the call for those who have come after her but also create a hypothetical phonebook to continue to help others . . . well, that's Elissa for you.

It is my hope that the term AYA continues to become more well known. It is my hope that if we continue to spread awareness and help those around us navigate this terrifying diagnosis, we will all benefit. Just like there is no "I" in team, I speak from experience when I say that we are stronger together.

If you are reading this, my guess is cancer has touched your life in some way, shape, or form. Please know that you are not alone.

Hey, Elissa, we got this.

CHAPTER TEN

WHAT DO YOU NEED?

When "Help" Isn't All That Helpful

From the very beginning, my goal was to communicate with you in a way that feels like you're reading about my journey in real time. And even though this is not a "cancer book," the progression of my disease does indeed have an impact on my narrative trajectory.

While I've been writing this book, my cancer has spread.

When friends and family learn of the progression of this disease (at this point it's only spread to my left breast), they are reaching out to express concern and to offer assistance, as friends and family do. But as the offers flow in, I am thrown back to those first days and weeks after receiving my original diagnosis.

Everyone wanted to help. Everyone wanted to send me something or buy me something or knit me something or make me something or even paint me something that would make me happy and help take the sting out of a suddenly crappy change in direction that my life had just taken.

It makes me very proud to realize how much more proficient and precise I have become about communicating my needs and responding to the constant stream of offers that are beginning to roll in. I know they all come from a place of love and support—and now I know how to speak up for myself to ensure I get the right kind of support from everyone.

It's that beautiful silver lining showing up again, even in the midst of my cancer's progression. Today, as opposed to when I was first diagnosed, I know myself on a deeper, more intimate level. Today my inner strength and resolve have been fortified. Today my life is rich, resonant, and without fear, which allows me to stand toe to toe with this disease no matter where it goes or what it does.

I have grown and charted completely new territory since my diagnosis, but *I am still me.* The essence of me remains unchanged.

What has changed, though, is how I relate to my cancer. Now I can verbalize my needs and desires without preamble or apology—and I have even created a platform that allows the other thrivers to do the same.

When I was first diagnosed, the offers came in fast and furious; they were a constant hum in my ear: *How can I help? What can I get you?* **What do you need?** Usually, my answer was something vague and indistinct, such as, "I don't really need anything. The fact that you're reaching out is more than enough for me!"

My guess is that when people heard my nebulous, nonspecific response back then, they probably reacted in a couple of different ways.

- They either breathed a sigh of relief and thought, *Whew! I'm off the hook! Thank goodness I don't have to go any further down this rabbit hole because I'm definitely out my depths with this scary cancer thing!*

or

- They sent me gifts anyway, of their choosing, which was well meaning . . . but also the reason I ended up with thirty blankets, fifteen scented candles, and more pillows, perfumes, and pretty little doodads than I could count.

It's not that a blanket is a bad choice for a gift. I love blankets! But even as someone who likes to be cozy, thirty was way more than I needed. My point is that if you're looking for a gift to share with someone who has cancer, there's a more efficient way to fill that gap and honor the recipient's preferences. Get them something that you know they need.

Unfortunately, the raw truth about receiving "cancer gifts" that you don't necessarily want or need is that it creates an additional burden. We don't have the time or energy to be sorting through stuff that doesn't really fit our needs. Now in addition to getting to chemo, making my daughter's lunch, and remembering to take my meds, I have to figure out how to store thirty blankets, fifteen candles, seven knickknacks, and a partridge in a pear tree.

Not only is nonspecific gift giving burdensome to the patient (well, to *me*, anyway, and I know for a fact that plenty of other cancer patients share this point of view), but it can also come across as insensitive because the gift giver isn't taking the recipient's needs or desires into account at all.

The process of searching for and selecting an appropriate gift for someone with a chronic or terminal illness (and I'm speaking from my personal experience with this terminal illness stuff) is uncomfortable and unsettling. It's not like shopping for a wedding or birthday or Christmas gift. It can whip up all kinds of latent, deep-set emotions, and it often brings the gift-giver closer to their own mortality than they care to be. *It stirs stuff up.* I realize this.

When people insist on giving gifts that they've chosen themselves, they are often—not *always* but often—using it to soothe their own fear or address their own deep-set insecurity. It shouldn't be the patient's responsibility to make sure everyone around them (the well-meaning gift giver included) feels more comfortable about cancer. Your fears are yours to bear. We've got enough on our plate.

This is precisely why I created a cancer gift registry: to create a direct line between a patient's unique, specific needs and a gift giver's heartfelt desire to help. WeGotThis.org is all about filling these gaps, providing creative solutions, and offering options that will make it easier on everyone. There's no reason why one person should receive thirty blankets.

Why not take the guesswork out of giving? Why not go to a registry and get precisely what the patient has already identified as a need or a desire? Why take a wild guess at what you think the patient might want, when nine times out of ten, your selection is based on what *you* think they need rather than what they actually want?

The Gift of Specificity

I'll always remember the first "cancer gift" I received as a direct result of my having asked for it *specifically*. It made me feel like my preferences and desires really mattered and like my voice was really being heard.

As part of my preparation to begin my very first round of chemo, I wanted to cut my hair short before I would lose it. So when my friends Dean McDermott and Tori Spelling texted me asking if there was anything that I needed before chemo started, I had a real answer for the first time. This was in the middle of the pandemic, and I wasn't comfortable going to a hair salon. I needed someone to come to my house, trust that they had been careful, and wouldn't get me sick before I started treatment. Within an hour after telling Dean and Tori what I needed—really needed—I had someone booked to come to my house and cut my hair. She's still my hairdresser to this day.

Even as I was gazing out of our living room window while my full, healthy hair was falling to the floor in tiny little piles, and even though I was receiving this haircut in preparation for my first round of chemo, which was a really crappy thought, I still remember thinking, *Thank you, thank you, thank you, Tori and Dean. Thank you for caring enough to give me exactly what I needed.*

That they recommended this top-notch hairstylist was certainly gift enough in and of itself. That they sent her to my home was icing on the cake. But when I went to pay her for her services and she refused, telling me that everything had already been taken care of (compliments of Tori and Dean), I didn't know quite what to do.

Even though I'd fully expected to pay for this service myself, I still remember feeling so comforted and *taken care of.*

That's why our gift registry brings such value to so many. It gives patients a chance to choose the products they want—the stuff that will bring them the most happiness—and it gives gift givers the opportunity to fill those needs in a highly specific way, with no guesswork involved!

I post a regular feature on Instagram called "We Got Recs," where I select different products I've used in my daily life and demonstrate why I find them practical and useful. I like to post my own candid feedback on products that patients may want and need throughout treatment. It's a great way to showcase some of the products and services that I actually enjoy.

Here is a quick list of a few of the coolest products that I recommend (if anyone making a registry needs ideas to start their own):

Elissa's Top Five Favorite Things to Register For

Note: These items do not appear in order of preference or priority. It's just a simple list of some of the stuff I happen to like and happen to use in my own life.

1. **The Nonsense of Nosebleeds:** Most cancer patients who have undergone chemo know that nosebleeds are definitely a "thing," but fear not. There's a

product called Nampons™ that's specifically designed to stick right up your nose! It expands for gentle pressure and contains a gentle clotting agent to stop nosebleeds. Similar in form and function to, well, let's just say the product name I'm thinking of rhymes with the word "Nampon". . .

2. **Took Take:** There are a lot of great solutions for remembering which pills you took or need to take, and I met a fellow thriver who came up with one of my favorites. Her product sticks right to the medicine bottle, and you pull off the tabs each time you're supposed to take your pills. Pillboxes can be a great solution, too, but I've found that there are many medications that aren't intended to be mixed with other pills. Each pull of the tab is like the benefit of Eric texting me to make sure I took my pills.

3. **Bombas Socks:** Snuggly, warm, and super well made, this seamless sock doesn't rub against the toes. As someone who has had many cuticle infections throughout chemo, this distinction of no seams in the toes makes a huge difference in my daily comfort.

4. **Crocs:** Slip them on and off without having to bend down and without even having to get out of your chair during chemo! Great for swollen feet or if you're dealing with neuropathy. Comfort to the feet when comfort is what's needed most! My feet never go far without Crocs.

5. **Flipmits:** These three-in-one gloves are a great solution for cold hands while also having options for function. They act as fingerless gloves, fold over into mittens, or roll down to be sweatbands. I love products that can be helpful during chemo but that I could also use on a run or something not at all cancer related. I like using Flipmits if I am in a type of chemo that I would ice my fingertips to prevent neuropathy. The rest of my hand can stay warm while I freeze the rest. Definitely not the intention of the product, but the founder, Matt, is brilliant and a huge supporter of our cancer community.

You might ask: what kinds of things belong in someone's gift registry or cancer wish list? The answer is very simple: whatever they want.

I have been told by fellow thrivers that they feel totally comfortable registering for things that are more medically related, such as barf bags or wigs. But they would feel uncomfortable registering for things that were simply to bring them joy or comfort. The words "selfish" or "needy" were used as concerns of how they didn't want to feel.

People who are supporting you through your treatment want you to be happy. They want you to feel comfort and joy. I know this for a fact from the thousands of supporters I encounter throughout my personal life and through the nonprofit. It is so essential to remember that we are not just cancer patients. We are also humans.

Throughout chemo there are many days where we feel incredibly sick or incapable of doing the simplest things. But in between treatments, we usually get a period where our symptoms subside before the next round begins, and we get to feel good. Feeling like our "normal" selves kind of good.

I understand the feeling of guilt during this time because I felt it. Everyone is showering you with love and support, and on some days, you feel totally fine and like you don't need that support. But if you're honest with yourself, you know that most days you do need it and that you absolutely deserve to still be showered with love on the days that you don't. I deserved the date nights with my husband when I could handle being seated upright at a restaurant. I deserved the outing at Universal Studios when we needed to feel like kids again. I deserved to feel like myself whenever I possibly could, and you absolutely do, too.

CHAPTER ELEVEN

DON'T FORGET TO DANCE

Life Lessons

I have cancer, and it sucks.

The experience of living with cancer has taught me plenty of important lessons, many rooted in the undeniable fact that I have been forced to live with this disease.

But every insight I have shared—every principle about life and living that I have put forward in the pages of this book—is both relevant and instructive on a larger, more universal scale.

You don't have to have cancer to practice the principles we have explored. You only need to have within you the passion and the will to embrace life as fully as you can. To cherish every moment. To take control of the things you can control. To understand that "winning" is something that *you* have the ability to define (and redefine, if necessary). That you can do more than merely survive in this world: *You can thrive.*

Even though life itself is a serious pursuit, never take yourself so seriously that you forget to have fun.

Put simply,

Never, ever forget to dance.

Even if you're facing the trial of a lifetime (say, terminal cancer), don't forget to dance.

While we are alive in this world, we owe it to ourselves to try to live our very best lives. To balance the serious with the whimsical. To seek joy and find happiness.

For me, this means singing my favorite songs, eating my favorite foods, hanging out with my favorite people, providing a platform and a resource that helps other cancer thrivers live their very best lives, and dancing with my daughter and my husband every night to bring the day to a close.

There's a balance, of course: Life is not all about the dance. I also get chemo regularly, eat healthy food, drink lots of water, take my medicine at the appointed times (thank you again, Eric!), and live responsibly so that I can, well, continue to live.

I want to make the intentional effort to create as many great days as I have crappy days and to create as many moments of joy as I have moments of pain and discomfort. More, if I can manage it. Certainly, there is a lot about the disease of cancer that I cannot control, but there are also many things I can control. I *can* bring this balance into my life—not all the time but much of the time—and being able to maintain this balance is what keeps me feeling connected, grounded, and purposeful.

This is why I work hard to not only create happy encounters and meaningful moments but to also capture those moments in a way that allows me to swing back to them again and again whenever I feel like it. Cancer has taught me how to create some of the best days and the brightest moments I've ever had in my life, and for that, I am grateful. The icing on the cake is that I can return to those moments whenever I want to, by writing them down in a note on my phone called "Best Days" and plucking them from my memory whenever the mood hits me.

The "Best Days" are days that will remain in my heart and mind forever. I am grateful that I had sense enough to write down the details while they were still fresh. This way they remain lucid and alive, even when the passage of time tries to blur their edges. I return to them often, on good days, on boring days, but especially when I'm feeling low, sick, or discouraged.

I'm honored to share a few of my reflections with you here. They are proof that even when you're facing trials and tribulations, life is simply, and awesomely, beautiful.

Best Day in Santa Barbara

On this day Eric and I decided to go all out. I was feeling very sick and down from the chemo. But on this day I refused to let it get the best of me. It doesn't always happen this way. I'm not Superwoman, able to fling off the disabling side effects of chemo with a simple shrug, but on this day I was able to push through my pain and discomfort.

We set out on a spur-of-the-moment but very-well-planned road trip. We were in need of olive oil and vinegar, which we had been consuming in mass quantities while starting to grow our own organic salads and veggies. I'm not going to dive into nutrition here, but when you're diagnosed with cancer, there's a fear that everything is trying to murder you. Needless to say, I wasn't buying store-bought salad dressings at this time.

Normally we just pick these items up from the local market. But on this day we decided to treat ourselves to the best oil and vinegar that Central Coast, California, could offer. We researched a few of the spots where they had the best of the best and then hopped in the car for a beautiful forty-five-minute drive to Santa Barbara.

The air was fresh and the experience unforgettable. We started the morning with the perfect breakfast sandwiches and mochas from one of our favorite spots, then headed to the beach to just walk around. After that we headed to another great spot to grab the best tacos we've ever eaten.

Okay, if it sounds like we got a little sidetracked from our original mission of getting olive oil and vinegar, that's because we *did* get a little sidetracked . . . which was one of the best parts. We did pick up the olive oil and vinegar, too, though! We just took our sweet time.

Why was this one of my best days? It represented one of the first times since being diagnosed that we'd gifted ourselves with life's most precious commodity: *time.* We embarked on this road trip early in my cancer journey, which really helped set the stage and lay the groundwork for how we developed and nurtured this healthy mindset moving forward. Namely, that when you want to do something, do it.

Best Day of Golf

We were in the process of launching WeGotThis.org, and I was planning our first in-person fundraiser—a golf tournament in my hometown of Andover, Massachusetts. I'd never planned anything like this, and the fact that I only had about twelve weeks to plan an event that normally takes the pros a minimum of six months to a year to organize pushed the stakes up even higher.

We'd already raised about $100,000 from a GoFundMe campaign we'd launched earlier, so awareness was beginning to grow, and I was fairly confident that we'd get a good turnout.

My goal going into this fundraiser was to try to raise about $10,000, $15,000 at the most; $20,000 was pretty much a pipe dream, but I kept it in the back of my mind anyway, just in case we got really, really lucky.

The good news: On the day of the event, we had a swarm of volunteers who pitched in to help. The bad news: A few weeks *before* the event, I found out there were tumors in my brain.

Here we'd planned everything down to its most minute detail, then something unplanned—like brain tumors—pop up out of nowhere. Bummer.

About a week before the tournament, I found myself receiving a five-day course of radiation, completely unexpected.

Plenty of well-meaning people urged me to cancel the fundraiser. They encouraged me to "take it easy" and to "put myself first." Little did they know that, in my life, moving forward with the projects and priorities that are most important to me is one way I *do* take care of myself.

My doctor had already told me that the decision to proceed or not to proceed was, ultimately, mine, which afforded me an important measure of additional control.

And control is exactly what I took.

The tournament was a groundbreaking success. We maxed out at 144 golfers, and we had over 200 people at the dinner. People I hadn't seen since high school came out to support. Everyone knew my story, and everyone was willing and happy to help.

I didn't hit the original goal of $10,000.

I *exceeded* it—ten times over. We raised $100,000 that day.

Chemo, radiation, and all other unexpected setbacks be damned.

Why was this one of my best days? It made me realize I had been underestimating my capabilities. The event itself helped me develop more of a growth mindset, which set our nonprofit on a similar trajectory. WeGotThis.org has become so much larger than I'd ever imagined, so much more impactful and resonant throughout the entire cancer community. I cannot and will not sell my nonprofit short. I had a $10,000 idea that was actually a $100,000 idea. Its meteoric rise has only just begun, and I will do everything in my power to ensure its continued growth.

Best Day with My Siblings

I had just started a new chemo regimen after discovering a recurrence in my breast and some new tumors in my brain, and I was feeling very, very low, physically and emotionally.

We started by driving out to the Malibu Pier. It's the same drive I take to get to my chemo, so it doesn't seem like it would elicit the happiest of emotions, *but it did*. My stepsisters' presence lifted my spirits and pulled me out of the darkness. Again, chemo, be damned.

We hit all my favorite places on this day, one of the best days in my life: lunch at a happy, healthy place called the Malibu Farm; coffee at one of my favorite spots in the world, Café 27, which happens to be on the side of a cliff; and dessert at Inn of the Seventh Ray, a tranquil oasis that fills me with inner peace.

On the drive home, we pulled into a lookout point and just stood together in comfortable silence, looking out over the water, soaking it all in.

That evening we swung back home and snatched up Eric, and we all headed to dinner at Castaway in Burbank, a beautiful bird's-eye-view restaurant that overlooks the valley and all of LA.

I ended that day feeling better than I had in a long time. In the course of only a few hours, I'd hit all my favorite spots, with all my favorite people. On this gloriously transformative day, two awesome women, whom I referred to as my stepsisters, became something else. We were always close, but I was specific in the accurate term of stepsisters up until this trip. I now just call them my sisters.

A happy addendum: While I was writing this book—just a few days ago, in fact—I was feeling low, listless, and painfully uncertain about my own future. So I decided to take this same "road trip" again, this time by myself. With a frown on my face (very rare for me), I forced myself behind the wheel, took those beautiful routes, and hit the spots we'd visited years earlier.

And by the end of my solo road trip, my despair had dissipated. My grief and uncertainty had lifted. I'd taken control of my darkness by driving directly to the light, directly to the places that had made me happy and brought me joy. And it worked.

But the day spent with my sisters was what created the memory in the first place. How lucky I am to have shared that experience with them! How fortunate I was to have been present enough to write it down so that these scenes can remain alive and vivid. How cool it was to be able to retrace my steps, going solo this time, and use it as a tool to help lift me up when I was feeling low. And how magnificent it was to nurture and deepen my relationship with two women who I care for so deeply.

Why was this one of my best days? In a single day, we hit so many of my favorite places. We could have gotten breakfast, coffee, lunch, and dessert all in one place. This was the first time I realized that we could just take our time. We laughed. We talked. We cruised along the Pacific Coast Highway.

On this special day, I even redefined my relationship with silence. Those wordless moments when the three of us stood together on the lookout, soaking in the view, were every bit as precious as our joyous conversations. They lifted me up. They helped propel me past my own pain and discomfort.

Best Day . . . on a Game Show!

Let's Make a Deal was preparing to tape a special episode dedicated to breast cancer awareness, and after a rigorous interview process by the show's producers, Eric and I were selected to be contestants.

In the hours leading up to the taping, I was so sick I didn't know whether we'd even be able to make the drive to the studio. But once I felt the energy of the audience—and the kind, compassionate energy of the show's host, Wayne Brady—I felt great! The fog of nausea and discomfort had suddenly lifted. (I don't ever remember experiencing such a sudden cessation of sickness in my life, in fact. Ever.)

Wayne Brady was awesome. After calling me down from the audience to stand beside him—cameras rolling and me, almost hyperventilating with excitement—he asked me to talk about WeGotThis.org and what we were all about. This was not only extremely validating, but I'm pretty sure it was also the first time I'd spoken publicly—and to such a large audience—about the organization. Everything about the entire experience felt surreal.

Believe it or not, Eric and I ended up winning the Big Deal of the Day, which is everything you could possibly win! Everything behind Door #1, Door #2, *and* Door #3 was ours! I literally felt like I was going to faint.

Part of this grand prize included a trip to New Zealand, but we decided later (a few weeks after we got home) to forego this part of the prize simply because it would have been a bit too ambitious a trip for us, given the circumstances.

Believe it or not, giving up New Zealand wasn't a bummer for us at all. I *still* felt like a winner! I had gone on national television for a game show that I had watched for years, and I was the big winner. That once-in-a-lifetime experience alone truly was the prize.

In fact, turning down New Zealand helped me redefine what victory looked like; it helped me expand my understanding of "winning." I didn't need a trip to New Zealand to prove that I'd emerged as the winner of the day! *I knew I won.* I knew that that moment was ours and could never be taken away. And I knew that the memory itself would remain with me forever.

Why was this one of my best days? I was a contestant on *Let's Make a Deal* with my husband standing right at my side in a matching costume! And because I didn't let the fact that I wasn't well enough to make the trip to New Zealand prevent me from feeling like a winner!

After the show, Wayne autographed the giant Noggin Boss hats that Eric and I were wearing. He wrote, "Eric, you're married to a champ."

I love that he wrote that and I can't deny that I am indeed a champ, but he forgot one important fact: *I'm* married to a champ, too!

Best Day of Dancing

This is how the ritual started: I had just gotten home one day when Eric met me at the door wearing the biggest smile and said, "Come right this way! I want to show you something!"

He had made a video while I was out and couldn't wait to show it to me.

The video showed Eric holding our daughter Ellie (then only weeks old) in his arms, dancing to the song "It Would Be You" by Ben Rector.

I watched, through tears of happiness and gratitude, Little Baby Ellie. Swaying in her daddy's arms, enjoying the sounds of Ben Rector and the rhythm of the music.

That's how it all began.

That very same day, we started having dance parties in our house. It's become our nighttime ritual: In the same way that making sure your children brush their teeth or wash their face every night before they go to bed, *we make sure we dance together.* Every single night.

Fast-forward from that special day to *this* day, and Ellie can dance on her own now. She even has her own lovely, eclectic taste in music. Sometimes we dance to her favorite artists like Britney Spears, Journey, Lady Gaga, and of course, Taylor Swift.

Why was this one of my best days? It established a regular rhythm and a beautiful end-of-day ritual for the three of us. What could be better than having a dance party every night as a way to bring the day to a close?

That first day, when Eric played the video that showed he and Ellie dancing, our sweet little girl was just a babe in his arms. But today she is an active participant. She *chooses* to dance with her mommy and daddy every night, and I'm deeply proud of the fact that we taught her this wonderful ritual. I'm proud of the fact that she values the joy this rhythmic ritual gives her, and I love that she knows how to express this joy on her own now, without our prompting.

A happy sidenote: Not too long ago, we met the musician Ben Rector, and we had the chance to tell him that his music and his song, "It Would Be You," launched a family ritual that we still honor to this very day. (He was very flattered.)

We dance together because we like to. We dance together because we love music. We dance together because, well, it's *fun*.

This dancing scene puts us on the perfect path toward the conclusion of this book because it lets me return to some essential wisdom I really want you to take with you.

Life is short. Life is precious. We are not meant to simply survive life. As fully engaged and fully empowered human beings who can choose how we embrace this thing called life, we must also learn to thrive each and every day, each and every moment, even during the dark days.

Before I had cancer, my goal in life was never to simply "survive." If someone asked me how my day was going and it wasn't that great, my response would be, "Eh, I'm surviving." So if that was how I describe a not-so-great day before, why would that be my goal now? Should the bar be lower because I have cancer?

My goal is to thrive. I want to live life to the fullest, not just stay alive. I don't feel like a thriver every day. We are all human and have our ups and downs, with or without cancer.

For me, fighting cancer is only half the battle.

Ensuring a rich quality of life is the other half—and it's way more fun!

Our time on this earth is finite and limited. We are not built to last forever. We are all terminal. Eventually, we all *fall asleep*.

But as long as we're awake and alive and pulling breath into our lungs, let's play the music loud and enjoy the rhythm as much as we possibly can.

As long as we're living, let's *live*.

Before we fall asleep . . .

Don't forget to dance.

ACKNOWLEDGMENTS

I would like to express my deepest gratitude to everyone who has supported and helped bring this book to life.

To Kristin Clark Taylor, thank you for helping me breathe life into my stories. Pulling from all of my life's memories was a monumental undertaking, and I'm so grateful to have done it with you by my side.

To my fellow thriver, Sarah Fischer, thank you for running the final laps with me and ensuring that I communicated everything I wanted to share with my audience. You captured who I am and how I want to be heard, and I cannot thank you enough.

To my incredible team at WeGotThis.org—Sarah Kovacs and Amber Packer—your dedication, hard work, and collaborative spirit have propelled my life's mission forward. Sarah, if it weren't for your sincere investment of time, love, and energy into this project, I truly don't believe it would have come together as it did. I will forever be grateful to work alongside you.

WeGotThis.org would not exist without the tireless efforts of my dear friends Paris and Frank Hill. There were moments when I couldn't get out of bed, yet you kept the wheels turning, allowing us to release the first nonprofit gift registry for cancer patients. You will forever hold a monumental place in the heart of WGT.

To everyone who has donated to WeGotThis.org, your generosity has made a real impact, and I am profoundly grateful for your contributions to support our cancer community.

A heartfelt thank you to my talented designer, Becca Levian at Skye High Interactive. Your creativity and vision brought this project to life in ways I never imagined. I'm so grateful you were part of WeGotThis.org from its earliest stages—when it was just a crazy idea I was brainstorming from bed.

Naren, I don't think it was a coincidence that we kept running into each other during my first ImpactEleven event. I wouldn't have taken this giant leap without your confidence and guidance. Thank you to Lauren and the entire Amplify team for your passion and dedication to this project. You worked with my whole story and gave it the time and attention it deserved.

Billye (www.billyedonya.com), you have always seen me so much deeper than just the surface, and I've felt that in every picture you've taken of me and my family. You've brought so many powerful visuals of our community to life. I treasure your images, your lifelong friendship, and your unwavering support.

Ethan (www.ethanpines.com), thank you for photographing my true self. You brought my individuality as an author to life and captured the essence of how I hope people see me.

To my alma mater, Babson College, thank you for equipping me with the tools and mindset to pursue my dreams and for being an enduring part of my life, long after graduation.

Dr. Marla Lipsyc-Sharf, your quality of care means more to me than you will ever fully know. You're not only keeping me alive, but you're doing so while prioritizing my ability to live a comfortable, fulfilling life. I am forever grateful.

A special thank you to my parents, whose love, guidance, and support have shaped me into the person I am today. Mom, as we always say, we are a team, and we're always stronger together. While my cancer isn't genetic, I know my strong will and eagerness to help others were passed down from you. Dad, thank you for embracing how much I keep you on your toes. The reflections and stories we share are woven throughout the pages of this book. To my stepdad, Les, and my stepmom, Denise: I love you both and am so grateful that my life has been enriched by having you in it.

To my in-laws, Bruce and Arlene Kalver, my first personal encounter with cancer as an adult came through both of you. Arlene's relentless fight with stage 4 lymphoma showed me that our diagnosis doesn't define our outcome. You are a true inspiration, and I'm in awe of your continued strength. Watching Bruce's caregiving role provided me with my first insight into what it means to be a caregiver up close. I cannot thank you both enough for showing me what love, strength, and hope look like in action.

Finally, to my incredible husband, Eric, thank you for your unwavering love, patience, and encouragement. Your belief in me has been a constant source of strength, and I wouldn't want to live this life without you by my side.

ABOUT THE AUTHOR

At 34, Elissa Kalver was diagnosed with Stage IV Metastatic Breast Cancer just before her daughter's first birthday. Refusing to simply survive, she launched WeGotThis.org—the world's first nonprofit cancer gift registry—during her 5th round of chemo. The platform allows cancer thrivers to request the items they truly need and gives loved ones a meaningful way to support them.

Elissa's story and outlook inspire others to shift their mindset, motivating growth, resilience, and connection in individuals and organizations alike. Her experience redefined success and strengthened her inner fight, leaving audiences inspired, confident, and determined to find their own path to success.

Learn more at wegotthis.org